MEDITERRANEAN DIET
MEAL PREP COOKBOOK

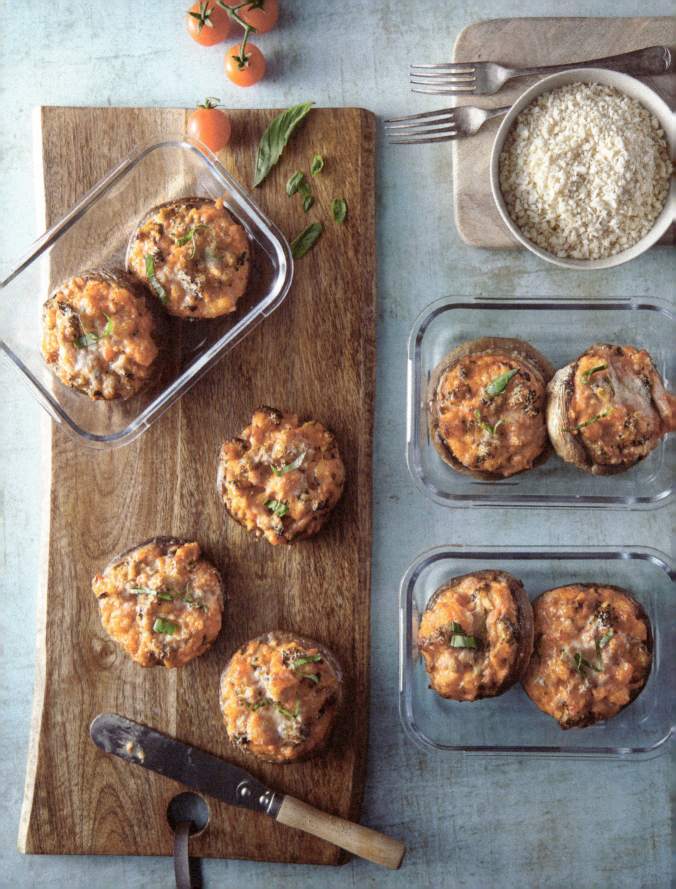

MEDITERRANEAN DIET
MEAL PREP
COOKBOOK

Weekly Plans and Recipes for a Healthy Lifestyle

LINDSEY PINE, MS, RDN, CLT

Photography by Darren Muir

ROCKRIDGE PRESS

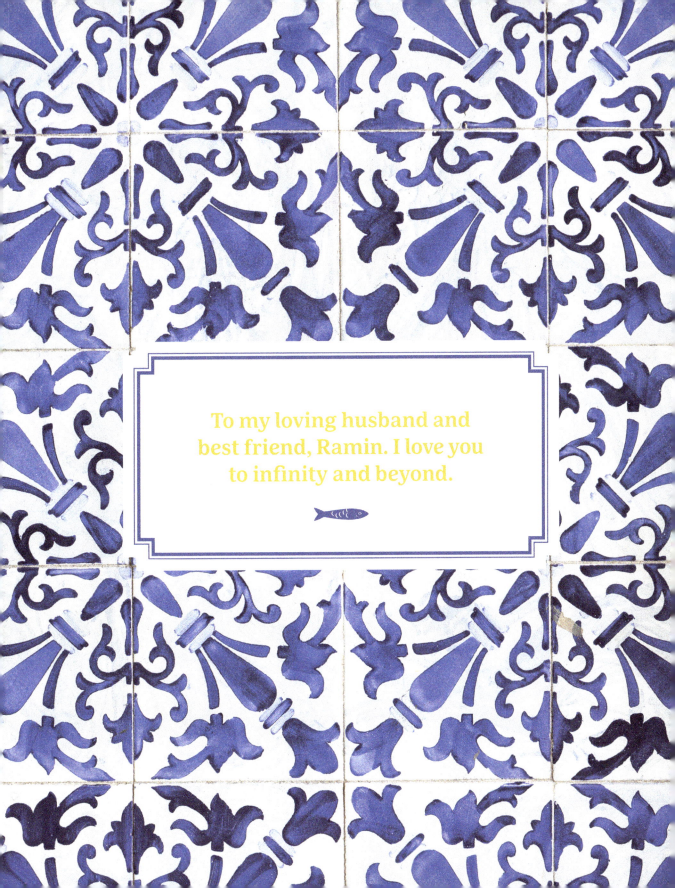

To my loving husband and
best friend, Ramin. I love you
to infinity and beyond.

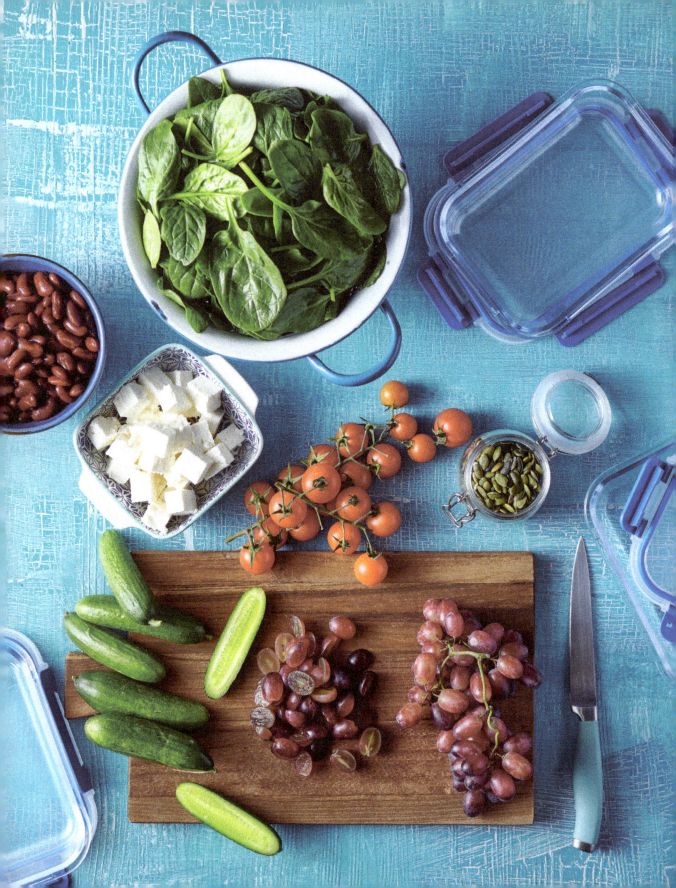

Contents

Introduction

I was a huge fan of the Mediterranean diet before I ever knew there was an official style of eating called the Mediterranean diet. While attending culinary school and working in restaurants in Seattle from 1999 through 2001, I fell in love with food from Spain, the south of France, North Africa, Lebanon, Greece, Italy, and more. Dishes from these regions are packed with herbs, spices, olive oil, legumes, grains, vegetables, and tons of flavor. Traveling to areas such as Nice, the Cinque Terre, and Barcelona taught me to respect quality ingredients and treat them with simplicity.

Fast-forward to graduate school in Los Angeles, where I was studying to become a registered dietitian. I started doing research for my master's-degree project on the topic of food and mood, and an eating pattern called the Mediterranean diet kept popping up. The research supporting the benefits of this eating style was plentiful.

In mid-2019, my husband was diagnosed with heart failure, and the Mediterranean diet emerged once again while we discussed his necessary lifestyle overhaul. Not only is eating in a Mediterranean way delicious, but it's also a wonderful heart-healthy dietary pattern. Notice that I said dietary *pattern*. You will only reap the benefits of a healthy diet if it becomes a habit that is completely ingrained in your lifestyle. This is why I not only prepare this type of cuisine in our home, but I also do a lot of meal prep to make my life easier and give my family healthy food that can be reheated quickly.

In addition to caring for my family, I work a full-time day job and have a business on the side. I definitely have a lot going on in my life, and meal prepping allows me to actually focus more of my attention on work and family. It's the most amazing feeling to come home from the office and know that dinner is already made! It gives me more time to get in a good sweat session at the gym after work, and then my husband and I have more time to spend together in the evenings. Better yet, breakfast and lunch for the next day are already made too!

It excites me not only to share my favorite style of cooking with you, but also to share it in a way that will ultimately save you time, reduce food waste, and support your physical and mental health. How wonderful it is that we have the opportunity to nourish ourselves and our families with delicious flavors that can also improve our overall well-being!

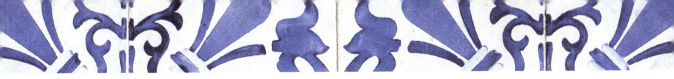

In this book, we'll cover the guiding principles of the Mediterranean diet, as well as meal prep basics, storage and container suggestions, shopping lists, and food-safety suggestions, with many tips and tricks incorporated into the recipes.

I hope you come away with the understanding that making the Mediterranean diet convenient is key to making sure we follow it and that home cooking and meal prep do not need to be difficult. In this book, I've included six weeks' worth of meal preps where I will remove the guesswork for you by providing exact servings for exact recipes. Once you have learned these recipes and techniques, the possibilities for additional weekly meal preps are practically endless. Consequently, the book also includes tons of bonus recipes so that you can customize your own meal prep menus! Let's get cooking!

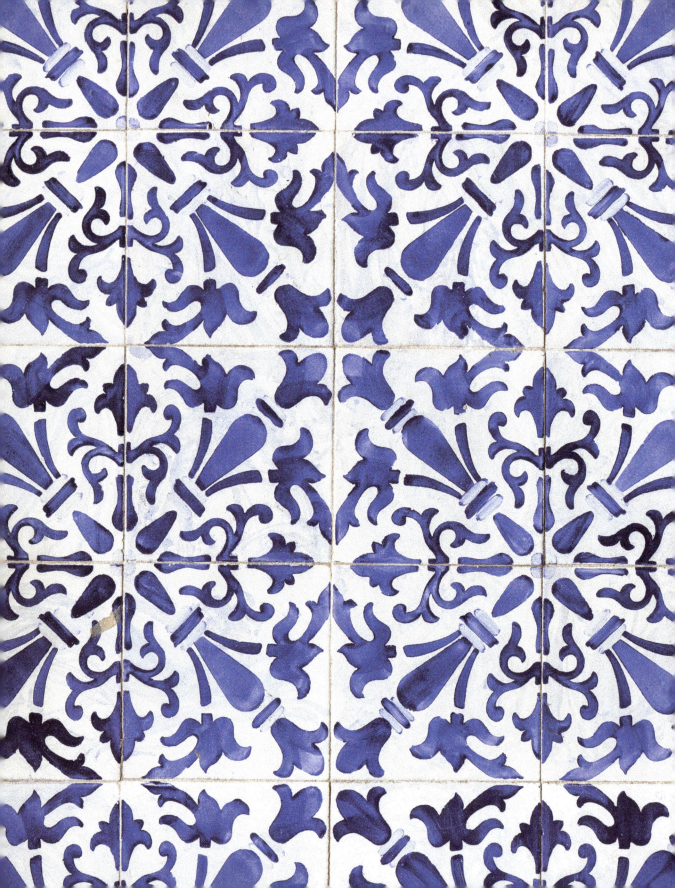

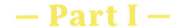

— Part I —

Mediterranean Diet 101

Before we get to the food, it's important to really understand what makes up the Mediterranean diet and how to enjoy it through an easy meal prep lifestyle. The aspect of *lifestyle* is a key ingredient, because the Mediterranean diet isn't just about food (and some wine); it also emphasizes eating meals and spending time with friends and family, which is incredibly important for our emotional health, mindfulness, and self-care. This diet encourages you to appreciate food, develop physical fitness, and enjoy life.

Although spending a few hours in the kitchen to meal prep on the weekend may not scream "family time," overall, you'll actually end up spending less time in the kitchen during the week. That means you'll have more quality time with your loved ones, more time to get that fitness routine in after work, and more time in general to do something that makes you happy.

After explaining the ins and outs of what the Mediterranean diet is, including the health benefits and the best types of foods to eat, we'll go into detail about meal prepping techniques and guidelines that will set you up for success. Included is information about essential equipment and storage containers that you'll need, plus grocery-shopping tips, and the dos and don'ts of food safety and storage.

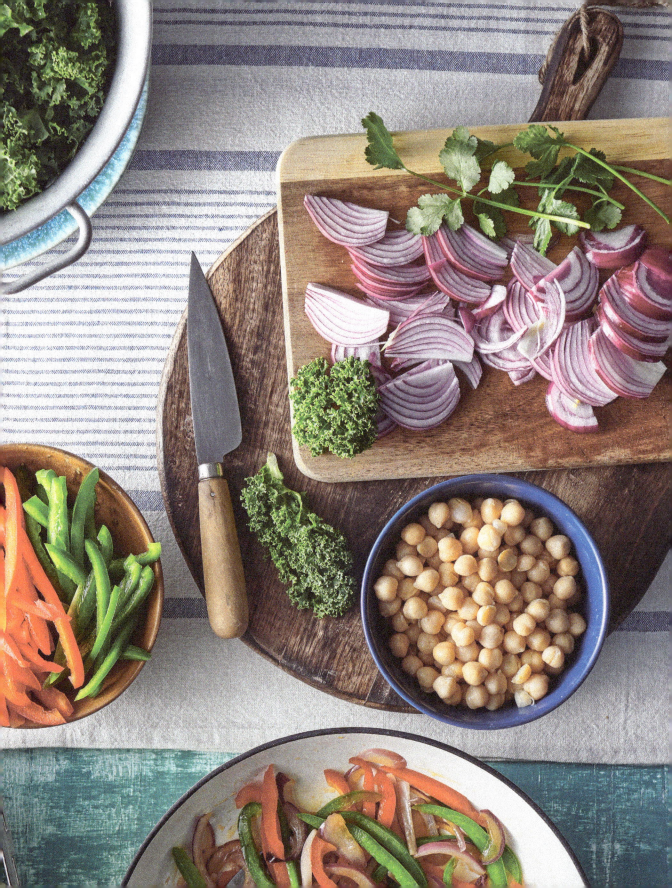

CHAPTER 1

The Mediterranean Philosophy

When we say "Mediterranean *diet*," we're not necessarily talking about weight loss. The original Greek meaning of the word "diet" actually refers to a way of living. That said, the Mediterranean diet is definitely *not* a fad weight-loss regimen where you will starve yourself, count calories, buy expensive products, or exclude entire food groups. Rather, it's a lifestyle that you have to immerse yourself into beyond just the food you eat.

The Mediterranean diet was first defined in the 1960s based on researchers' observations of what people ate in Greece and Southern Italy, where residents were seemingly healthier compared to Americans and northern Europeans. Since that initial study, much more research has been conducted to show the numerous health benefits of eating the Mediterranean way.

There may not be a set of strict rules when following a Mediterranean eating style, but there is a set of guiding principles regarding the types of foods you should eat more and less of. The principles do not specify concrete amounts of food to eat. Instead, this is a dietary pattern that is balanced and sustainable for the long haul. The great thing about it is that you get to make this dietary pattern fit your lifestyle.

The Guiding Principles

The Mediterranean diet draws on flavors from all the countries that border the Mediterranean Sea, giving us many types of fresh, quality ingredients to work with and ensuring that we won't get bored. The key to following this way of life can be defined by the following principles:

Focus on plant-based foods. The bulk of this diet consists of vegetables, fruits, herbs, spices, whole grains, legumes, nuts, and seeds. Your meals should be built around these foods.

Cook with healthy fats. Olive oil reigns supreme, but healthy unsaturated fats may also come from nuts, seeds, and avocados.

Eat fish/seafood at least twice per week. Seafood and fish give us heart- and brain-healthy omega-3 fatty acids. Good sources include salmon, tuna, mackerel, trout, sardines, and herring.

Consume eggs, dairy, and poultry in moderate amounts. The term "moderate" is subjective. These items can be incorporated daily, but don't make them the center of the plate for every meal. Dairy will most often be eaten in the form of yogurt or cheese.

Limit consumption of red meat and sweets. Think of these items more as treats. The Mediterranean diet includes a relatively low amount of the saturated fat found in red meat, which is why red meat is limited. Instead, opt for leaner protein, such as chicken and turkey.

Drink red wine—in moderation. Moderation with wine means up to one five-ounce glass per day for women and two for men. But if you don't already drink, it's not required that you start.

Your main beverage should be water. Hydrate with water instead of sugary beverages. Coffee and tea are okay, but ditch the sweeteners.

Engage in physical activity daily. Whether you prefer walking, dancing, or spending time at the gym, move your body each day.

Make social time a priority. Spend time with friends and family, including sharing meals together.

The Health Benefits

While the exact mechanisms for improved health are not 100 percent clear, researchers believe that the health benefits of this dietary pattern may come from high amounts of fiber, antioxidants, vitamins, minerals, phytonutrients (chemicals naturally found in plants that have health benefits), and healthy unsaturated fats taking the place of saturated and trans fats. It is also believed that ingesting this variety of nutrients has an anti-inflammatory effect in the body. It's truly amazing how components in food work synergistically, creating more benefit together than alone. The Mediterranean diet may help prevent myriad chronic diseases, since it can do the following:

REDUCE THE RISK OF HEART DISEASE

This dietary pattern can reduce cholesterol, protect cells against damaging oxidative stress, and lessen inflammation and platelet aggregation, helping reduce the risk of America's number one killer.

IMPROVE COGNITIVE FUNCTION

Reducing inflammation and oxidative stress may help slow the aging process of the brain and even protect against cognitive decline, including Alzheimer's disease.

PREVENT AND CONTROL TYPE 2 DIABETES

High intake of fiber and low intake of sugar through eating minimally processed plant foods can help control blood-sugar levels and improve insulin sensitivity.

POSSIBLY PROTECT AGAINST SOME FORMS OF CANCER

The plant-based foods of the Mediterranean diet contain very powerful tumor-growth-inhibiting, anti-inflammatory compounds, including lycopene from tomatoes, ferulic acid from whole grains, and organosulfurs (phytonutrients found in cruciferous vegetables that may protect against cancer) from onion and garlic.

IMPROVE GUT MICROBIOME

The bacteria in the gut affect many bodily functions, including immunity, weight maintenance, and cognition. Fiber from the Mediterranean diet feeds our good bacteria, which in turn produce gut-healthy, short-chain fatty acids that may prevent common inflammatory conditions, such as obesity, type 2 diabetes, and heart disease.

Mediterranean Diet Pyramid

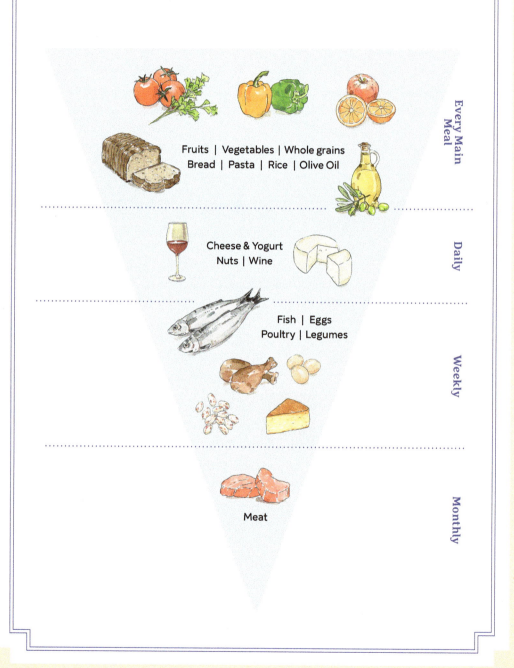

Fruits | Vegetables | Whole grains
Bread | Pasta | Rice | Olive Oil

Every Main Meal

Cheese & Yogurt
Nuts | Wine

Daily

Fish | Eggs
Poultry | Legumes

Weekly

Meat

Monthly

Eating healthy, whole, and minimally processed foods can result in weight loss even if you aren't intentionally counting calories. Plus, weight loss aids in almost all the health benefits mentioned on page 5.

Feed the Lifestyle

Vegetables, fruits, whole grains, legumes, nuts, seeds, olive oil, and olives are plentiful in the Mediterranean lifestyle and make up the backbone of the diet. Another key component of the Mediterranean diet is seafood, which is a very important source of the omega-3 fatty acid that most people who eat a standard American-style diet don't get enough of. Overall, the focus is on whole, seasonal, and fresh items, but it's perfectly fine to take some shortcuts by using quality canned, jarred, and frozen items, such as canned fish and beans, frozen berries, and jarred artichokes and roasted peppers. Plain Greek yogurt, cheese, eggs, and poultry are scattered throughout the dietary pattern, with red meat showing up the least.

You may be happy to know that a moderate amount of red wine is included in the Mediterranean lifestyle, but water is generally the preferred go-to beverage. If the idea of drinking plain old water with every meal doesn't appeal to you, try infusing your water with herbs and fruits for a burst of flavor. Coffee and tea are definitely acceptable, but try to limit added sweeteners.

FOODS TO EAT

The following foods are all components of the Mediterranean diet:

- Vegetables
- Fruits
- Onions and garlic (including garlic or onion powder)
- Legumes, such as beans, chickpeas, soybeans, lentils, and dried peas
- Tofu and tempeh
- Potatoes and sweet potatoes
- Whole grains, such as whole-wheat pasta, whole-wheat breads, quinoa, brown rice, bulgur, and farro
- Herbs and spices
- Salt and pepper
- Extra-virgin olive oil
- Avocados
- Peanuts and nuts, such as walnuts, almonds, pistachios, and pecans

- Seeds, such as sesame, sunflower, pepitas (green pumpkin seeds), flax, hemp, and chia
- Fish and seafood, such as salmon, tuna, sardines, mackerel, herring, shrimp, clams, and mussels (canned is okay)
- Eggs
- Plain Greek yogurt
- Cheese, such as feta and Parmesan
- Jarred antipasti-style items, such as roasted red peppers, capers, olives, and artichoke hearts packed in olive oil
- Condiments, such as mustard, pesto, and hot sauce
- Turkey and chicken
- Beef, pork, and lamb (eaten in moderation)
- Red wine
- Water
- Unsweetened coffee and tea

FOODS TO AVOID

Try to avoid the following foods as much as possible:

- Ultra-processed foods: You can usually identify these types of foods through very long ingredient lists that include additives, artificial flavors, added colors, and sugar.
- Trans fats
- Processed meats, such as hot dogs and lunch meats
- Refined grains and pasta
- Excess added sugars from pastries, candies, and table sugar
- Sugar-sweetened beverages

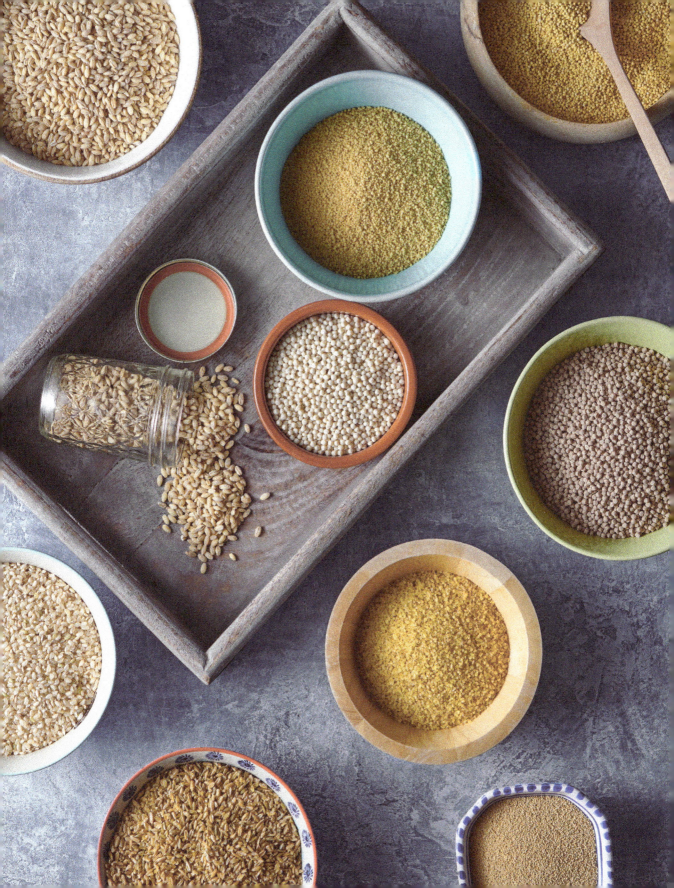

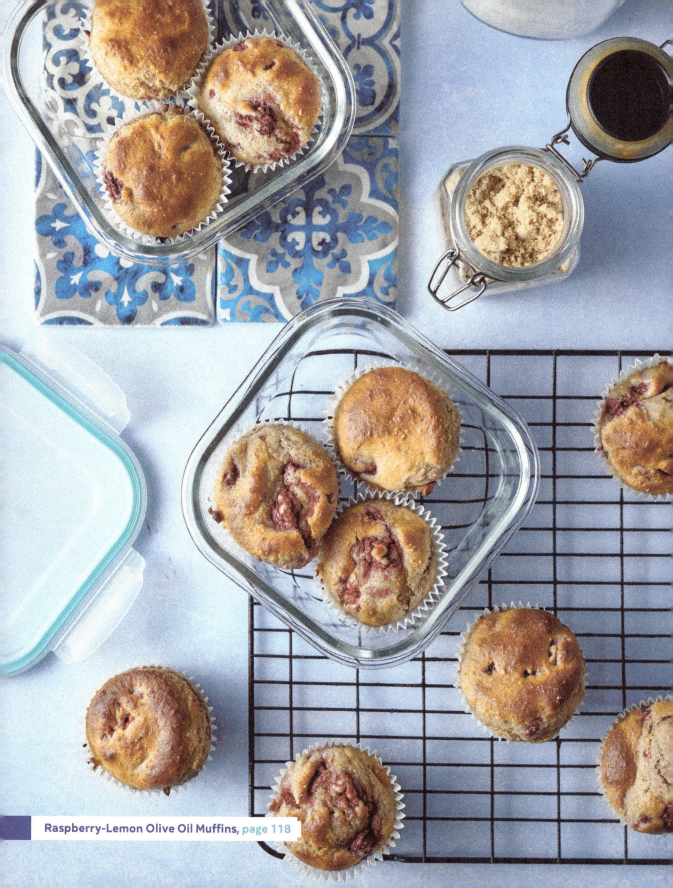

Raspberry-Lemon Olive Oil Muffins, page 118

CHAPTER 2

The Art of the Prep

The benefits of meal prepping for a Mediterranean diet lifestyle are plentiful. Some of my favorites include:

Portion control. By planning your portions ahead of time, you'll avoid overeating. That's automatic calorie control without counting calories!

Balanced meals. The Mediterranean diet is already a very balanced way of eating, and meal prep will take that idea even further because you won't be buying random food out of convenience. Your balanced meal will be right at your fingertips.

Save time in the kitchen. Think about all those times when you get home from work and cringe at the idea of having to make dinner. With meal prep, when you get home after a long day, you can simply heat up your food.

Less stress at the grocery store. You'll be in and out of the grocery store more quickly, because you will have a list of everything needed for your meals.

Save money. Going out to eat is expensive, especially when you factor in tax and tip, and even the gas to drive to the restaurant. You will save tons of cash just by eating at home. Plus, when you shop from a list, unnecessary items that aren't part of your recipes won't end up in your shopping cart.

Cut down on food waste. When you know what you're making for the week, you will actually use what you buy. There will be no more buying too much and then having to toss out what isn't used.

You will have more time overall. The Mediterranean diet emphasizes physical fitness and being social with friends and family. Because you'll be in the kitchen less, you'll have more time to devote to those activities.

Meal Prep Basics

The terms "meal planning" and "meal prep" are often used interchangeably, but they are actually quite different. Meal planning is nothing more than figuring out what you're going to make and when you're going to eat it throughout the week. Meal prepping takes this a step further: It involves cooking multiple days' worth of food over the course of a few hours and portioning out the food into single-serving containers to be eaten throughout the week. Successful meal preppers are those who plan ahead!

If you're new to meal prepping, start slowly by prepping two or three recipes and building on that prep in the weeks that follow. Now let's go over some helpful dos and don'ts to start your meal prep journey.

DOS

- ☑ **Do get organized and develop a game plan before grocery shopping.** Write that plan down and set yourself up for success! This also includes making sure that you have the appropriate cooking equipment.

- ☑ **Do change the menu each week.** You don't want to get bored with eating the same food every week. Plus, a healthy diet is built upon a variety of foods and nutrients.

- ☑ **Do choose recipes that utilize different cooking methods, including the stovetop, oven, and even no-cook recipes.** For example, if all your recipes require the oven, chances are everything won't fit in the oven at the same time, which means you will waste time.

- ☑ **Do purchase airtight containers in a variety of sizes.** The last thing you want is spilled food all over your car or lunch bag.

- ☑ **Do portion out meals into individual containers as soon as you finish preparing them.** Finish what you started!

☒ **Don't choose complicated recipes.** If you choose difficult recipes, you'll probably be less likely to continue prepping each week. Simple can still be delicious.

☒ **Don't wait until the last minute on Sunday night to start prepping.** Instead, shop on Saturday and prep on Sunday, or try shopping and chopping veggies on Saturday and completing the meal prep on Sunday.

☒ **Don't cook without checking your container supply.** Make sure you have enough of the right kind of containers.

☒ **Don't assume that prepped food will last in the refrigerator forever.** Most prepared foods will keep for about five days.

☒ **Don't start prepping with a sink full of dirty dishes.** Prep will go more smoothly if you start with a clean kitchen.

Storage Solutions

You can't meal prep without containers to store the finished product. There are a few factors to think about when choosing containers, including size, shape, material, and cleanability. Weight is also an important factor, especially if you have to transport a bag of filled containers to the office. In addition to choosing the right types of storage containers, don't forget to purchase the right quantity. There are so many containers on the market, so which ones should you buy? Let's look at the various types:

CONTAINER TYPES

BPA-free plastic. Be sure the label states that the product is BPA (Bisphenol A)-free, as well as microwave- and dishwasher-safe. Plastic containers are the lightest and most convenient, but they can hold on to smells even after the container has been washed.

Glass. Glass containers are naturally BPA-free. They can also withstand wear and tear, and they can go into the microwave, oven, and dishwasher. The downsides are the heavier weight and higher cost than plastic, and the fact that glass is breakable.

Leakproof. Make sure that your containers and lids are leakproof. Trust me on this one!

Grocery Shopping Tips

With thousands of products at the grocery store, roaming the aisles for healthy foods that are within your budget can be intimidating. Here are my top tips for navigating the aisles:

1 Shop the whole store, not just the perimeter. There are so many healthy foods throughout the inner aisles that will be missed if you only shop the perimeter.

2 Canned fish like salmon, tuna, and sardines are great budget-friendly options. Choose either water-packed products or those packed in olive oil.

When buying fish at the seafood counter, look for fish surrounded by crushed ice. The fish should not smell fishy, and the flesh should look firm and not mushy.

3 Shop for grains, nuts, seeds, and dried fruits from the bulk bins, when possible, to save money and limit your purchase to just the amount you need.

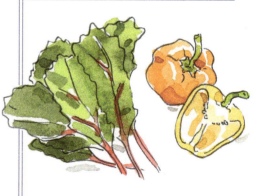

4 Large chain international supermarkets often sell produce for significantly less money than typical American supermarkets.

5 **Pick up some chopped jarred garlic.** It saves time, and you won't get the garlic smell on your hands.

Garlic and onion powders save time when you don't want to chop aromatics. This works well when you're using the onion and garlic for seasoning purposes only, rather than adding bulk to a dish, such as for a stew.

6 **Frozen fruits and veggies are just as nutritious as fresh.** Frozen fruits are great for smoothies and for topping chia pudding, oats, and yogurt. You'll also find edamame in the frozen-food aisle.

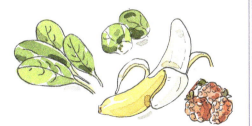

7 **Buy tomato paste in resealable tubes,** not in those little cans.

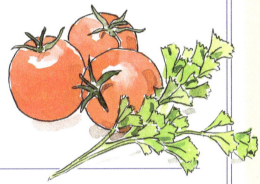

8 **Canned beans and tomatoes are great convenience items.** Look for reduced-sodium, low-sodium, or no-salt-added products if you are watching sodium intake.

If you have extra storage space in your home, buy larger quantities of canned items like tomatoes and beans at bulk discount stores.

Various sizes and numbers of compartments. Depending on what you're prepping, sometimes you'll want different shapes and sizes. For example, be sure to get some small dressing containers and smoothie cups. Some containers, called bento boxes, have dividers that come in handy if you don't want foods to touch.

Bags. Sometimes a bag may be most suitable for fruit or trail mix. A more environmentally sustainable alternative to a plastic baggie is a reusable silicone food bag.

FOOD STORAGE GUIDELINES

The topic of food storage isn't exactly the most exciting part of cooking, but it's necessary if we want to stay safe from food-borne illness. In the restaurant world, we practice something called FIFO, or first in, first out. By placing the oldest use-by date in the front, we'll ensure that we're using the oldest product first, which will help us use all our food before it goes bad and cut down on food waste.

Don't keep cold or hot foods sitting out for more than two hours. We don't want to keep food in the temperature "danger zone" of 40 to 140°F for more than that amount of time. If the temperature of the environment is over 90°F, the rule of thumb is one hour maximum. It's as simple as keeping your hot foods hot and your cold foods cold.

To cut down on cross-contamination, place all your uncooked meats on the bottom shelf of the refrigerator and your ready-to-eat foods toward the top. Make sure all foods are covered or wrapped well.

Check the temperature of your refrigerator, which should not go above 40°F. Your freezer should be set to 0°F.

Grab a label maker and label the containers that go into the freezer. If you don't have a label maker, use a permanent marker to write on a piece of masking tape, which you can then place on the container. Have you ever unwrapped a freezer item not knowing what it was or when it was put there? This eliminates the problem! Items in the freezer last a long time, but they won't last forever. Label each item, writing what it is and a use-by date.

Use the following handy chart as a guide to how long food will stay at peak quality in the refrigerator and freezer. Just remember, though, no matter what the perishable opened item or prepared item is, be sure to throw it away after seven days.

	Refrigerator	Freezer
RAW BEEF, LAMB, AND PORK CUBES, STEAKS, AND ROASTS	3 to 5 days	4 to 12 months
RAW GROUND MEATS	1 to 2 days	3 to 4 months
RAW POULTRY	1 to 2 days	9 months
FRESH, RAW FISH	1 to 2 days	2 to 3 months
UNCOOKED TOFU	7 days	5 months
SOUPS AND STEWS	3 to 4 days	2 to 3 months
COOKED DISHES WITH MEAT, EGGS, POULTRY, OR FISH	3 to 4 days	2 to 3 months
COOKED BEANS	6 to 7 days	6 to 12 months
COOKED GRAINS	4 to 6 days	6 months
YOGURT (WITHOUT ADD-INS)	1 to 2 weeks	1 to 2 months (only use for smoothies or baking, since texture will change)
SALADS: EGG, PASTA, CHICKEN, FISH	3 to 4 days	Not recommended
HARD-COOKED EGGS	7 days	Not recommended
MUFFINS	3 to 7 days in the pantry	2 to 3 months

Source: FoodKeeper App (a collaboration between the USDA's Food Safety and Inspection Service, Cornell University, and the Food Marketing Institute)

Reheating and Thawing

Thawing. Never leave food on the counter or on top of the refrigerator overnight to thaw. Your grandma may have done this back in the day, but this is a great way to get sick!

The first choice for thawing food is to let it thaw in the refrigerator. The bigger the item, the longer it will take to thaw. Some items can take up to a few days, so plan ahead. If you didn't plan ahead, you can also defrost food in the microwave, as long as you use that food right away. Smaller items can be defrosted under a stream of cool running water in the sink, but I'm not a huge fan of this method, because it wastes water.

Reheating. When reheating any previously cooked food, you must bring the internal temperature of the thickest part of the dish up to 165°F. Because all microwaves are different, play around with the cooking times to ensure your food is heated to a safe temperature.

Equipment

You don't need cupboards full of fancy, expensive equipment to cook great food; you just need the basics. Luckily, the equipment needed for meal prepping isn't any different from the items you probably already have in your kitchen. You don't have to go in for the latest and trendiest equipment, but certain essential items will definitely make cooking easier.

MUST-HAVE

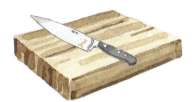

Sharp 8- or 10-inch chef's knife. This is my number one essential item. Your knife is like an extension of your arm. Not only will a dull knife drive you crazy when you're trying to chop, but dull knives are also more dangerous than sharp ones.

Large cutting board. Choose a couple of 18-by-12-inch polypropylene or wood boards. It's helpful to have separate boards for produce and meat.

18-by-13-inch sheet pan and silicone baking mat (or parchment paper). The baking mat or parchment paper will make cleanup faster.

Skillet. Because meal prep includes more than one serving, I use a 12-inch nonstick pan most often to ensure I'm not overcrowding the pan.

Glass or ceramic baking dish. Get yourself a 9-by-13-inch dish, an 8-by-11-inch dish, and a 9-by-9-inch dish. These types of dishes are often sold in sets.

Heat-proof spatula. This is a great tool for stirring and scraping bowls and pans.

Blender. A good-quality blender is helpful for making smoothies and sauces.

Mixing bowls. Have a variety of sizes on hand, including mini-prep, 1-, 2-, 3-, and 5-quart bowls. Glass, ceramic, or stainless steel will work fine.

Measuring spoons. Standard sets include six sizes. It can be handy to have two sets.

Measuring cups for dry and liquid ingredients. It's best to have standard sets of metal or plastic cups for dry ingredients, as well as 2-cup and 4-cup glass liquid measuring cups that can be used in the microwave to heat liquids.

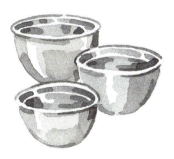

Food Substitutes for Those with Allergies

If you have a food allergy or sensitivity, try the following substitutes and read the manufacturer's suggestions. For example, both Bob's Red Mill and King Arthur Flour offer gluten-free baking tips on their websites.

 Milk. Unsweetened, nondairy, plant-based beverages such as almond, cashew, or soy milk. Soy milk contains significantly more protein than nut-based beverages.

 Cheese. There are many very good plant-based cheeses on the market. Some are even pre-shredded! A few popular brands that make plant-based cheese are Daiya, Miyoko's, Kite Hill, and Follow Your Heart.

 Olive oil. Avocado oil

 Nuts or peanuts. Pumpkin or sunflower seeds

 Nut or peanut butter. Sunflower seed butter

 Grains containing gluten, such as farro, bulgur, and pasta. Quinoa, millet, and gluten-free pasta

 Wheat flour. There are many good gluten-free baking flour blends on the market. Bob's Red Mill and King Arthur Flour are a couple of brands that make quality gluten-free flours specifically for baking.

 Eggs. Replace eggs in baked goods with a flax "egg." Mix 1 tablespoon ground flaxseed with 3 tablespoons water in a small bowl. Allow to thicken in the refrigerator for 15 minutes. Use 1 flax "egg" for 1 real egg in baked goods like pancakes and muffins.

 Red meat. If you don't eat red meat at all, feel free to use poultry instead.

Soy. In a recipe calling for edamame, use canned beans, such as white, pinto, black, or kidney beans or chickpeas.

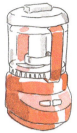

Food processor. Though it's not totally necessary, if you have one, you'll find you use it often to make Mediterranean sauces and dips such as pesto, Spanish romesco, and hummus.

Slow cooker. There's no need for a fancy model. A 6-quart cooker with high and low settings will do the job.

Citrus zester. A rasp type is also useful for finely grating cheese.

Paring knife. A sharp 3½-inch knife comes in handy for deveining shrimp, segmenting citrus, and many other tasks. A serrated paring knife is great for slicing tomatoes.

Outdoor grill and/or cast-iron grill pan for indoor grilling. An outdoor grill gives meat and veggies a great smoky taste, but if you don't have outdoor space or it's too cold to cook outside, an indoor grill is a terrific alternative.

Muffin tins. If you like baking muffins, then this item would be on the must-have list. Mini frittatas are trendy, too, but you can make a large frittata and cut it into slices instead.

What to Expect from Meal Plans and Recipes

Now that I've given you an overview of the basics of the Mediterranean diet and meal prepping, let's actually start cooking! I'm starting you off with six weeks' worth of meal preps, including grocery and equipment lists, order of operations to save the most time, and the recipes.

The Mediterranean diet doesn't include as much meat as other eating styles, so the amount of animal protein per serving may be a little less than what you're used to if you eat a typical American diet. With each prep, I've made sure to include one seafood dish.

After the six weeks of meal preps, you'll find 65 bonus recipes to create tons of other weekly meal prep combos. If a recipe within those six weeks of preps doesn't appeal to your tastes, feel free to substitute one of the bonus recipes.

I can't wait for you to get started on a new journey of wellness and delicious Mediterranean-style food!

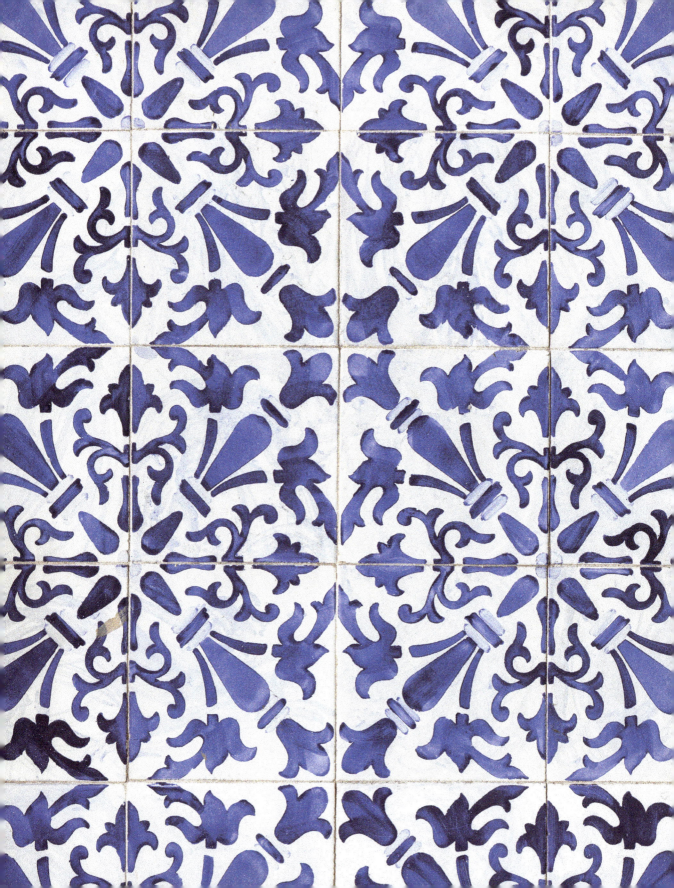

Part II

Meal Prep Plans with Recipes

Congratulations on taking the first step toward meal prepping! We'll start off with a smaller number of recipes over the next couple of weeks to ease you into the process. For weeks one and two, you'll make four recipes that include breakfast, lunch, and dinner, and then you'll increase to six recipes by week five, which will include breakfast, lunch, dinner, and a snack or sweet treat. Sometimes the snack can even double as a dessert.

Each meal prep includes a grocery-shopping and equipment list to make the whole process easier for you. To simplify the process even more, I've included step-by-step instructions so that you know the order of operations that will keep you in the kitchen for the least amount of time.

I'm a huge fan of balance, so each prep will also include a mixture of hot and cold items in addition to cooked and no-cook recipes.

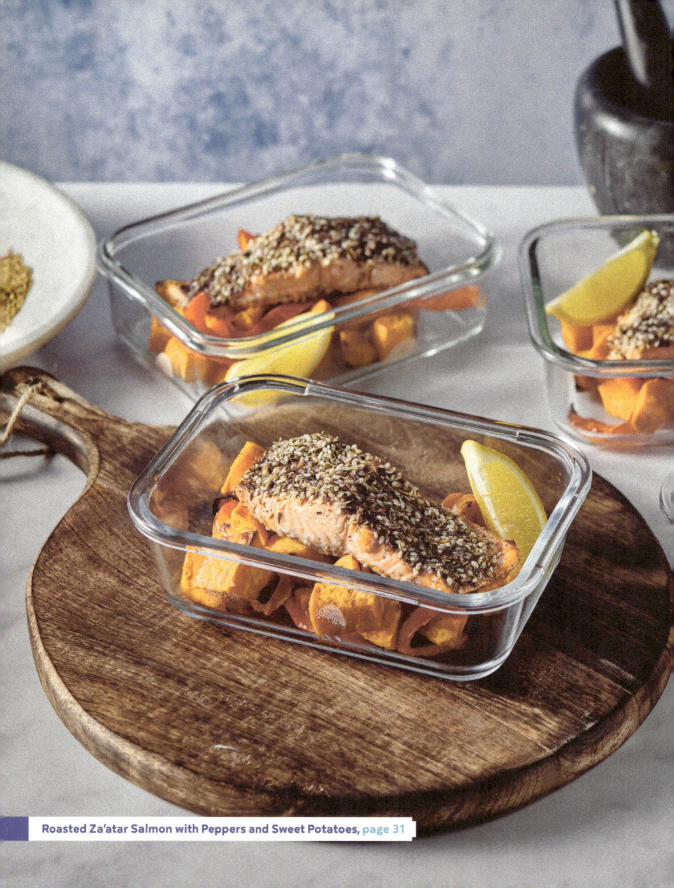

Roasted Za'atar Salmon with Peppers and Sweet Potatoes, **page 31**

CHAPTER 3

Prep 1

Meal prep 1 includes four meals to get you into the swing of things and set you up for success. You'll notice this prep involves a limited amount of chopping to make the first set of recipes even easier to prepare. While you'll have breakfast, lunch, and dinner covered, be sure to think of some grab-and-go snacks for an added boost of energy throughout the day and between meals. Items like fresh fruit, nuts, whole-grain crackers, and olives are a few no-cook items that are easily portable. If you make extra portions, feel free to freeze those for a later meal or incorporate them into your week as snacks.

Shopping List

PANTRY

- ☐ Chickpea flour (⅓ cup)
- ☐ Crushed tomatoes, 1 (28-ounce) can
- ☐ Dried Italian herbs
- ☐ Dried mint
- ☐ Dried thyme leaves
- ☐ Extra-virgin olive oil
- ☐ Garlic powder
- ☐ Kosher salt
- ☐ Onion powder
- ☐ Pure maple syrup (1 tablespoon plus 2 teaspoons)
- ☐ Sumac
- ☐ Vanilla extract (2 teaspoons)

FRESH PRODUCE

- ☐ Arugula, 1 (5-ounce) bag
- ☐ Carrots, shredded, 1 (10-ounce) bag
- ☐ Lemons (2)
- ☐ Mushrooms (4 ounces)
- ☐ Red bell peppers, large (2)
- ☐ Scallions (1 bunch)
- ☐ Spaghetti squash (3 pounds)
- ☐ Sweet potatoes (1 pound)

PROTEIN

- ☐ Eggs, large (2)
- ☐ Salmon fillet, skinless, boneless (1 pound)
- ☐ Turkey, lean (93%) ground (½ pound; freeze extra half if you can only buy a full 1-pound package)

DAIRY

- ☐ Greek yogurt, low-fat (2%), 1 (16-ounce) container
- ☐ Parmesan cheese, grated, 1 (5-ounce) container

GRAINS, NUTS, SEEDS, AND LEGUMES

- ☐ Almond butter, plain, unsalted (5 tablespoons)
- ☐ Almond milk, unsweetened vanilla (3⅓ cups)
- ☐ Almonds, sliced (½ cup plus 2 tablespoons)
- ☐ Chia seeds (3 tablespoons)
- ☐ Chickpeas, reduced-sodium, 1 (15-ounce) can
- ☐ Oats, old-fashioned (1⅔ cups)
- ☐ Sesame seeds (2¾ teaspoons)

OTHER

- ☐ Apricots, dried (⅓ cup)
- ☐ Sweet cherries, frozen (1⅔ cups)

Equipment

- ☐ Chef's knife
- ☐ Cutting board
- ☐ Measuring cups and spoons
- ☐ Mixing bowls
- ☐ Spatulas
- ☐ 2 (18-by-13-inch) sheet pans
- ☐ Silicone baking mats or parchment paper
- ☐ 12-inch skillet
- ☐ 8-by-11-inch glass or ceramic baking dish

Day	Breakfast	Lunch	Dinner
1	Cherry, Vanilla, and Almond Overnight Oats	Roasted Za'atar Salmon with Peppers and Sweet Potatoes	Carrot-Chickpea Fritters
2	Cherry, Vanilla, and Almond Overnight Oats	Turkey Meatballs with Tomato Sauce and Roasted Spaghetti Squash	Roasted Za'atar Salmon with Peppers and Sweet Potatoes
3	Cherry, Vanilla, and Almond Overnight Oats	Roasted Za'atar Salmon with Peppers and Sweet Potatoes	Carrot-Chickpea Fritters
4	Cherry, Vanilla, and Almond Overnight Oats	Turkey Meatballs with Tomato Sauce and Roasted Spaghetti Squash	Roasted Za'atar Salmon with Peppers and Sweet Potatoes
5	Cherry, Vanilla, and Almond Overnight Oats	Carrot-Chickpea Fritters	Turkey Meatballs with Tomato Sauce and Roasted Spaghetti Squash

Step-by-Step Prep

1. Begin by preheating the oven to 425° F and make the spaghetti squash for the **Turkey Meatballs with Tomato Sauce and Roasted Spaghetti Squash** (page 29).

2. While the squash is roasting, make the **Turkey Meatballs with Tomato Sauce** (page 29) and put them in the oven. Once the squash is tender, remove it from the oven, allow to cool, and scrape the flesh out with a fork. You will need that sheet pan for the next recipe.

3. Squeeze the lemon juice for the **Roasted Za'atar Salmon with Peppers and Sweet Potatoes** (page 31), **Carrot-Chickpea Fritters** (page 33), and **Garlic Yogurt Sauce** (page 165).

4. Prepare the peppers and sweet potatoes for the **Za'atar Salmon** (page 31) and set a timer for 10 minutes once they go into the oven. Remove the turkey meatballs when done and allow to cool.

5. Once the **Turkey Meatballs with Tomato Sauce** (page 29) are cool, place about 1 cup of spaghetti squash, 4 meatballs, and 1 cup of sauce in each of 3 containers and refrigerate.

6. Prepare the **Za'atar Salmon** (page 31) and place it in the oven with the peppers and sweet potatoes. Set a timer for 10 minutes for ½-inch-thick fillets or 15 minutes for 1-inch-thick fillets.

7. While the salmon and veggies are roasting, make the **Carrot-Chickpea Fritters** (page 33) mixture. Remove the salmon and veggies when the timer goes off and allow to cool. Once they are cool, divide the peppers, sweet potatoes, and salmon among 4 containers and refrigerate.

8. Cook the fritters and allow to cool once done. Make the **Garlic Yogurt Sauce** (page 165).

9. Once the **Carrot-Chickpea Fritters** (page 33) have cooled, place the arugula in 3 containers and spoon ¼ cup of the yogurt sauce into each of 3 sauce cups. Place 3 fritters in each of 3 separate containers (the fritters will be reheated later, while the arugula and sauce will not). Refrigerate.

10. Make the **Cherry, Vanilla, and Almond Overnight Oats** (page 35), spoon into 5 containers, and refrigerate.

Turkey Meatballs *with* Tomato Sauce *and* Roasted Spaghetti Squash

**MAKES
3 SERVINGS**

PREP TIME:
15 minutes

——

COOK TIME:
35 minutes

——

One of the best ways to add veggie goodness and stretch the amount of ground meat you have is to add chopped mushrooms. They also add flavor and moisture. Even if you don't like mushrooms, you'll never know they're in there.

FOR THE SPAGHETTI SQUASH

3 pounds spaghetti squash

1 teaspoon olive oil

¼ teaspoon kosher salt

FOR THE MEATBALLS

**½ pound lean
ground turkey**

**4 ounces mushrooms,
finely chopped (about
1½ cups)**

**2 tablespoons
onion powder**

1 tablespoon garlic powder

**1 teaspoon dried
Italian herbs**

⅛ teaspoon kosher salt

1 large egg

FOR THE SAUCE

**1 (28-ounce) can
crushed tomatoes**

1 cup shredded carrots

1 teaspoon garlic powder

1 teaspoon onion powder

¼ teaspoon kosher salt

TO MAKE THE SPAGHETTI SQUASH

1. Preheat the oven to 425°F and place a silicone baking mat or parchment paper on a sheet pan.

2. Using a heavy, sharp knife, cut the ends off the spaghetti squash. Stand the squash upright and cut down the middle. Scrape out the seeds and stringy flesh with a spoon and discard.

Continued »

Turkey Meatballs with Tomato Sauce and Roasted Spaghetti Squash *continued*

3. Rub the oil on the cut sides of the squash and sprinkle with the salt. Lay the squash cut-side down on the baking sheet. Roast for 30 to 35 minutes, until the flesh is tender when poked with a sharp knife.

4. When the squash is cool enough to handle, scrape the flesh out with a fork and place about 1 cup in each of 3 containers.

TO MAKE THE MEATBALLS AND SAUCE

5. Place all the ingredients for the meatballs in a large bowl. Mix with your hands until all the ingredients are combined.

6. Place all the sauce ingredients in an 8-by-11-inch glass or ceramic baking dish, and stir to combine.

7. Form 12 golf-ball-size meatballs and place each directly in the baking dish of tomato sauce.

8. Place the baking dish in the oven and bake for 25 minutes. Cool.

9. Place 4 meatballs and 1 cup of sauce in each of the 3 squash containers.

STORAGE *Store covered containers in the refrigerator for up to 5 days.*

TIP *Most packaged ground turkey comes in 1-pound packages. Because you only need ½ pound for this recipe, freeze the other half for a later time. The raw turkey can be frozen for 3 to 4 months.*

Per Serving: Total calories: 406; Total fat: 13g; Saturated fat: 5g; Sodium: 1,296mg; Carbohydrates: 45g; Fiber: 10g; Protein: 29g

Roasted Za'atar Salmon
with Peppers *and* Sweet Potatoes

MAKES 4 SERVINGS

PREP TIME:
10 minutes

———

COOK TIME:
25 minutes

———

Za'atar is a flavorful spice blend popular in countries such as Lebanon, Morocco, Tunisia, and Turkey. Sumac is a lemony, burgundy-colored spice found in the spice section of major supermarkets. If you're trying to cut down on salt, sumac is a great spice that adds tons of flavor.

FOR THE VEGGIES

2 large red bell peppers, cut into ½-inch strips

1 pound sweet potatoes, peeled and cut into 1-inch chunks

1 tablespoon olive oil

¼ teaspoon kosher salt

FOR THE SALMON

2¾ teaspoons sesame seeds

2¾ teaspoons dried thyme leaves

2¾ teaspoons sumac

1 pound skinless, boneless salmon fillet, divided into 4 pieces

⅛ teaspoon kosher salt

1 teaspoon olive oil

2 teaspoons freshly squeezed lemon juice

TO MAKE THE VEGGIES

1. Preheat the oven to 425°F.

2. Place silicone baking mats or parchment paper on two sheet pans.

3. On the first pan, place the peppers and sweet potatoes. Pour the oil and sprinkle the salt over both and toss to coat. Spread everything out in an even layer. Place the sheet pan in the oven and set a timer for 10 minutes.

Continued »

Roasted Za'atar Salmon with Peppers and Sweet Potatoes *continued*

TO MAKE THE SALMON

4. Mix the sesame seeds, thyme, and sumac together in a small bowl to make the za'atar spice mix.

5. Place the salmon fillets on the second sheet pan. Sprinkle the salt evenly across the fillets. Spread ¼ teaspoon of oil and ½ teaspoon of lemon juice over each piece of salmon.

6. Pat 2 teaspoons of the za'atar spice mix over each piece of salmon.

7. When the veggie timer goes off, place the salmon in the oven with the veggies and bake for 10 minutes for salmon that is ½ inch thick and for 15 minutes for salmon that is 1 inch thick. The veggies should be done when the salmon is done cooking.

8. Place one quarter of the veggies and 1 piece of salmon in each of 4 separate containers.

STORAGE *Store covered containers in the refrigerator for up to 4 days.*

TIP *Mediterranean food tends to use lemon juice in many recipes. Squeeze the lemon juice for all recipes into one bowl at the beginning of the prep, and then you can just scoop out what you need during the cooking process.*

Per Serving: Total calories: 295; Total fat: 10g; Saturated fat: 2g; Sodium: 249mg; Carbohydrates: 29g; Fiber: 6g; Protein: 25g

Carrot-Chickpea Fritters

MAKES 3 SERVINGS

PREP TIME:
15 minutes

——

COOK TIME:
10 minutes

——

This dish is inspired by flavors from Turkey. Carrots, dried apricots, and mint add a slight sweetness that complements the sharp scallions, savory chickpeas, and garlicky yogurt sauce. If you buy a 10-ounce bag of shredded carrots, use the leftover carrots in Turkey Meatballs with Tomato Sauce and Roasted Spaghetti Squash (page 29).

2 teaspoons olive oil, plus 1 tablespoon

3 cups shredded carrots

1 (4-ounce) bunch scallions, white and green parts chopped

1 (15-ounce) can low-sodium chickpeas, drained and rinsed

⅓ cup dried apricots (about 10 small apricot halves), chopped

1 teaspoon garlic powder

1½ teaspoons dried mint

⅓ cup chickpea flour

1 egg

¼ teaspoon kosher salt

1 tablespoon freshly squeezed lemon juice

1 (5-ounce) package arugula

¾ cup Garlic Yogurt Sauce (page 165)

1. Heat 2 teaspoons of oil in a 12-inch skillet over medium-high heat. Once the oil is hot, add the carrots and scallions, and cook for 5 minutes. Allow to cool.

2. While the carrots are cooking, mash the chickpeas in a large mixing bowl with the bottom of a coffee mug. (I find a coffee mug works better than a potato masher.)

3. Add the apricots, garlic powder, mint, chickpea flour, egg, salt, lemon juice, and cooked carrot mixture to the bowl, and stir until well combined.

4. Form 6 patties and place them on a plate.

Continued »

Carrot-Chickpea Fritters *continued*

5. Heat the remaining 1 tablespoon of oil in the same skillet over medium-high heat. Once the oil is hot, add the patties. Cook for 3 minutes on each side, or until each side is browned.

6. Place 2 cooled fritters in each of 3 containers. Place about 2 cups of arugula in each of 3 other containers, and spoon ¼ cup Garlic Yogurt Sauce into each of 3 separate containers, or next to the arugula. The arugula and sauce are served at room temperature, while the fritters will be reheated.

STORAGE *Store covered containers in the refrigerator for up to 5 days. Uncooked patties can be frozen for 3 to 4 months.*

TIP *Raw chickpea flour has a strong beany taste, but that taste goes away when the flour is cooked. Find it in the baking aisle with the alternative flours. Store it in your freezer to keep the opened bag fresh longer.*

Per Serving: Total calories: 461; Total fat: 17g; Saturated fat: 3g; Sodium: 393mg; Carbohydrates: 61g; Fiber: 15g; Protein: 21g

Cherry, Vanilla, *and* Almond Overnight Oats

MAKES 5 SERVINGS

PREP TIME: 10 minutes

——

Overnight oats are one of the easiest and healthiest make-ahead breakfasts! You also have the option of eating them cold or heating them up. The possibilities for flavor combinations are endless, but this recipe is especially delicious with the combination of cherries with vanilla and almonds. If you need to make them gluten-free, just use certified gluten-free oats.

1⅔ cups rolled oats

3⅓ cups unsweetened vanilla almond milk

5 tablespoons plain, unsalted almond butter

2 teaspoons vanilla extract

1 tablespoon plus 2 teaspoons pure maple syrup

3 tablespoons chia seeds

½ cup plus 2 tablespoons sliced almonds

1⅔ cups frozen sweet cherries

1. In a large bowl, mix the oats, almond milk, almond butter, vanilla, maple syrup, and chia seeds until well combined.

2. Spoon ¾ cup of the oat mixture into each of 5 containers.

3. Top each serving with 2 tablespoons of almonds and ⅓ cup of cherries.

STORAGE *Store covered containers in the refrigerator for up to 5 days. Overnight oats can be eaten cold or warmed up in the microwave.*

TIP *Mason jars work very well for storing individual servings of overnight oats.*

Per Serving: Total calories: 373; Total fat: 20g; Saturated fat: 1g; Sodium: 121mg; Carbohydrates: 40g; Fiber: 11g; Protein: 13g

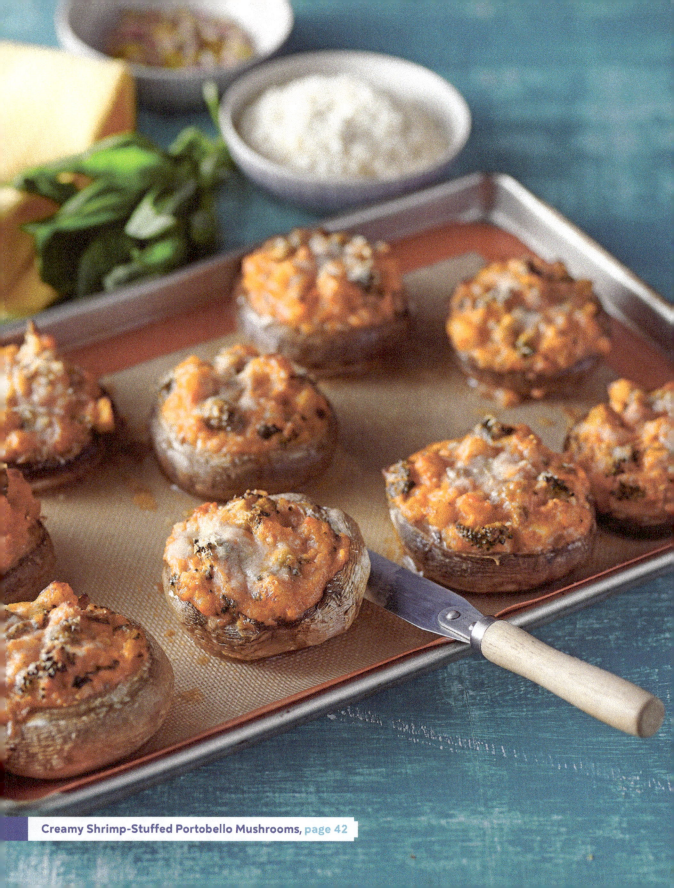

Creamy Shrimp-Stuffed Portobello Mushrooms, page 42

CHAPTER 4

Prep 2

Now that you have one prep under your belt, hopefully you feel extra confident this week to get in the kitchen and prepare four more recipes. You'll be making another breakfast and three lunch/dinner dishes, all with Italian flavors. With this week's prep, you'll use a variety of prepared ingredients that will ultimately save you time in the kitchen. Go easy on yourself and use these high-quality types of convenience foods. Not everything has to be homemade! Items like roasted red peppers, shredded cheese, precut broccoli florets, jarred chopped garlic, olives, panko bread crumbs, rotisserie chicken, and frozen shelled edamame can be game changers!

Shopping List

PANTRY

- ☐ Dijon mustard
- ☐ Dried rosemary
- ☐ Extra-virgin olive oil
- ☐ Honey
- ☐ Kosher salt
- ☐ Olives, black or kalamata (or other olive of your choice) (1 jar)
- ☐ Panko bread crumbs (¼ cup)
- ☐ Roasted red peppers (1 jar)
- ☐ Smoked paprika
- ☐ Sun-dried tomatoes, packed in olive oil (1 jar)
- ☐ Tomatoes, diced, no-salt-added, 1 (14.5) ounce can

FRESH PRODUCE

- ☐ Baby kale, 1 (5-ounce) bag
- ☐ Basil, fresh, 1 (½-ounce) container
- ☐ Broccoli florets, 1 (12-ounce) bag
- ☐ Chives, 1 (¾-ounce) bunch
- ☐ Fennel (1 bulb)
- ☐ Fresh fruit, 5 (1-cup) servings of your choice
- ☐ Garlic, chopped (1 jar) or head (1)
- ☐ Green apple (1 small)
- ☐ Lemons (2)
- ☐ Portobello mushrooms (6)
- ☐ Zucchini (2 medium)

PROTEIN

- ☐ Eggs, large (8)
- ☐ Rotisserie chicken (1 cooked)
- ☐ Shrimp, uncooked, peeled, deveined, frozen or fresh (10 ounces)

DAIRY

- ☐ Cheddar cheese, sharp, shredded, 1 (8-ounce) package
- ☐ Mascarpone cheese, 1 (8-ounce) container
- ☐ Milk, low-fat (2%) (½ cup)
- ☐ Parmesan cheese, grated, 1 (5-ounce) container (you should have enough left over from last week's prep if you made Prep 1)

GRAINS, NUTS, SEEDS, AND LEGUMES

- ☐ Edamame, frozen, shelled, 1 (12-ounce) bag
- ☐ Quinoa (1⅓ cup)
- ☐ Walnut pieces (3 ounces)

Equipment

- ☐ Chef's knife
- ☐ Cutting board
- ☐ Measuring cups and spoons
- ☐ Mixing bowls
- ☐ Whisk
- ☐ Spatulas

- ☐ 1 sheet pan
- ☐ Silicone baking mat or parchment paper
- ☐ 12-inch sauté pan or skillet
- ☐ 3½-quart saucepan
- ☐ 8-inch round cake pan or pie pan

Day	Breakfast	Lunch	Dinner
1	Broccoli, Roasted Red Pepper, Cheddar, and Olive Frittata with a side of fresh fruit	Rosemary Edamame, Zucchini, and Sun-Dried Tomatoes with Garlic-Chive Quinoa	Creamy Shrimp-Stuffed Portobello Mushrooms
2	Broccoli, Roasted Red Pepper, Cheddar, and Olive Frittata with a side of fresh fruit	Rotisserie Chicken, Baby Kale, Fennel, and Green Apple Salad	Rosemary Edamame, Zucchini, and Sun-Dried Tomatoes with Garlic-Chive Quinoa
3	Broccoli, Roasted Red Pepper, Cheddar, and Olive Frittata with a side of fresh fruit	Creamy Shrimp-Stuffed Portobello Mushrooms	Rotisserie Chicken, Baby Kale, Fennel, and Green Apple Salad
4	Broccoli, Roasted Red Pepper, Cheddar, and Olive Frittata with a side of fresh fruit	Rosemary Edamame, Zucchini, and Sun-Dried Tomatoes with Garlic-Chive Quinoa	Creamy Shrimp-Stuffed Portobello Mushrooms
5	Broccoli, Roasted Red Pepper, Cheddar, and Olive Frittata with a side of fresh fruit	Rotisserie Chicken, Baby Kale, Fennel, and Green Apple Salad	Rosemary Edamame, Zucchini, and Sun-Dried Tomatoes with Garlic-Chive Quinoa

Step-by-Step Prep

1. Preheat the oven to 375°F. Make the **Broccoli, Roasted Red Pepper, Cheddar, and Olive Frittata** (page 41).

2. While the frittata is in the oven, make the **Creamy Shrimp-Stuffed Portobello Mushrooms** (page 42).

3. Once the **Broccoli, Roasted Red Pepper, Cheddar, and Olive Frittata** (page 41) is cooked and removed from the oven, turn the oven down to 350°F. Allow the frittata to cool, then run a spatula around the outside and slide it out of the pan. Cut it into 5 pieces and place the pieces in 5 containers. Place 1 cup of fruit of your choice in each of 5 separate small containers or resealable bags. Refrigerate.

4. Bake the **Creamy Shrimp-Stuffed Portobello Mushrooms** (page 42). While they are baking, make the **Rosemary Edamame, Zucchini, and Sun-Dried Tomatoes** (page 44) and allow to cool.

5. Cook twice the amount of quinoa called for in the Garlic-Chive Quinoa recipe that goes with the **Rosemary Edamame, Zucchini, and Sun-Dried Tomatoes** (page 44). Once it is cool, set aside 2 cups of the cooked quinoa for the **Rotisserie Chicken, Baby Kale, Fennel, and Green Apple Salad** (page 46). Stir the chives into the remaining 2 cups of quinoa, then place ½ cup in each of 4 containers, along with the cooled edamame mixture.

6. Remove the **Creamy Shrimp-Stuffed Portobello Mushrooms** (page 42) from the oven and cool. Once they are cool, place in 3 containers and refrigerate.

7. Make the **Honey-Lemon Vinaigrette** (page 178). Make the **Rotisserie Chicken, Baby Kale, Fennel, and Green Apple Salad** (page 46). Divide the salad among 3 containers and place 2 tablespoons of vinaigrette in each of 3 sauce cups. Refrigerate.

Broccoli, Roasted Red Pepper, Cheddar, _and_ Olive Frittata

PREP TIME:
10 minutes

———

COOK TIME:
25 minutes

———

Frittata is simply a fancy-sounding word for an Italian-style open-faced omelet. They're great vehicles for adding tons of vegetables, especially on days when you need to clean out the refrigerator of veggie odds and ends. If you have leftover cooked rice or quinoa, you can add that to the dish as well.

Oil or cooking spray for greasing the pan

8 large eggs

½ cup low-fat (2%) milk

1 teaspoon smoked paprika

6 ounces broccoli florets, finely chopped (about 2 cups)

½ cup chopped jarred roasted red peppers, drained of liquid

⅓ cup pitted black olives, chopped (or other olive of your choice)

¼ cup shredded sharp Cheddar cheese, plus 2 tablespoons

1. Preheat the oven to 375°F and rub an 8-inch round cake or pie pan with oil, or spray with cooking spray.
2. Break the eggs into a large mixing bowl. Add the milk and smoked paprika, and whisk until well combined.
3. Add the chopped broccoli, red peppers, olives, and ¼ cup of cheese, and mix.
4. Pour the mixture into the oiled pan and top with the remaining 2 tablespoons of cheese. Bake for 20 to 25 minutes.
5. Once the frittata is cool, run a spatula around the sides and slice into 5 pieces.
6. Place 1 slice in each of 5 containers and refrigerate.

STORAGE _Store covered containers in the refrigerator for up to 5 days._

Per Serving: Total calories: 193; Total fat: 12g; Saturated fat: 5g; Sodium: 295mg; Carbohydrates: 7g; Fiber: 1g; Protein: 13g

Creamy Shrimp-Stuffed Portobello Mushrooms

MAKES 3 SERVINGS

PREP TIME:
15 minutes

—

COOK TIME:
40 minutes

—

Portobello mushrooms are great vehicles for all types of fillings. I've added some creaminess to this shrimp, broccoli, and tomato filling by adding some mascarpone cheese. Mascarpone is a silky smooth, slightly sweet Italian cheese—similar to cream cheese—and adds a luxurious richness.

1 teaspoon olive oil, plus 2 tablespoons

6 portobello mushrooms, caps and stems separated and stems chopped

6 ounces broccoli florets, finely chopped (about 2 cups)

2 teaspoons chopped garlic

10 ounces uncooked peeled, deveined shrimp, thawed if frozen, roughly chopped

1 (14.5-ounce) can no-salt-added diced tomatoes

4 tablespoons roughly chopped fresh basil

½ cup mascarpone cheese

¼ cup panko bread crumbs

4 tablespoons grated Parmesan, divided

¼ teaspoon kosher salt

1. Preheat the oven to 350°F. Line a sheet pan with a silicone baking mat or parchment paper.

2. Rub 1 teaspoon of oil over the bottom (stem side) of the mushroom caps and place on the lined sheet pan, stem-side up.

3. Heat the remaining 2 tablespoons of oil in a 12-inch skillet on medium-high heat. Once the oil is shimmering, add the chopped mushroom stems and broccoli, and sauté for 2 to 3 minutes. Add the garlic and shrimp, and continue cooking for 2 more minutes.

4. Add the tomatoes, basil, mascarpone, bread crumbs, 3 tablespoons of Parmesan, and the salt. Stir to combine and turn the heat off.

5. With the mushroom cap openings facing up, mound slightly less than 1 cup of filling into each mushroom. Top each with ½ teaspoon of the remaining Parmesan cheese.

6. Bake the mushrooms for 35 minutes.

7. Place 2 mushroom caps in each of 3 containers.

STORAGE *Store covered containers in the refrigerator for up to 4 days.*

Per Serving: Total calories: 479; Total fat: 31g; Saturated fat: 10g; Sodium: 526mg; Carbohydrates: 26g; Fiber: 7g; Protein: 26g

Rosemary Edamame, Zucchini, _and_ Sun-Dried Tomatoes _with_ Garlic-Chive Quinoa

MAKES 4 SERVINGS

PREP TIME:
10 minutes
—

COOK TIME:
15 minutes
—

Sliced sun-dried tomatoes in olive oil are a great convenience product and serve a dual purpose. Not only do you get the tomato strips, but you can also use the flavorful garlic-infused oil for cooking or adding to dressings. If you're not a rosemary fan, feel free to substitute a different herb such as oregano or basil, dried or fresh.

FOR THE GARLIC-CHIVE QUINOA

1 teaspoon olive oil

1 teaspoon chopped garlic

⅔ cup quinoa

1⅓ cups water

¼ teaspoon kosher salt

1 (¾-ounce) package fresh chives, chopped

FOR THE ROSEMARY EDAMAME, ZUCCHINI, AND SUN-DRIED TOMATOES

1 teaspoon oil from sun-dried tomato jar

2 medium zucchini, cut in half lengthwise and sliced into half-moons (about 3 cups)

1 (12-ounce) package frozen shelled edamame, thawed (2 cups)

½ cup julienne-sliced sun-dried tomatoes in olive oil, drained

¼ teaspoon dried rosemary

⅛ teaspoon kosher salt

TO MAKE THE GARLIC-CHIVE QUINOA

1. Heat the oil over medium heat in a saucepan. Once the oil is shimmering, add the garlic and cook for 1 minute, stirring often so it doesn't burn.

2. Add the quinoa and stir a few times. Add the water and salt and turn the heat up to high. Once the water is boiling, cover the pan and turn the heat down to low. Simmer the quinoa for 15 minutes, or until the water is absorbed.

3. Stir in the chives and fluff the quinoa with a fork.

4. Place ½ cup quinoa in each of 4 containers.

TO MAKE THE ROSEMARY EDAMAME, ZUCCHINI, AND SUN-DRIED TOMATOES

5. Heat the oil in a 12-inch skillet over medium-high heat. Once the oil is shimmering, add the zucchini and cook for 2 minutes.

6. Add the edamame, sun-dried tomatoes, rosemary, and salt, and cook for another 6 minutes, or until the zucchini is crisp-tender.

7. Spoon 1 cup of the edamame mixture into each of the 4 quinoa containers.

STORAGE *Store covered containers in the refrigerator for up to 5 days.*

TIP *When cooking veggies for meal prep, remember that they will continue to cook when you reheat your food, so don't overcook them the first time around.*

Per Serving: Total calories: 312; Total fat: 11g; Saturated fat: 1g; Sodium: 389mg; Carbohydrates: 39g; Fiber: 9g; Protein: 15g

DAIRY-FREE • GLUTEN-FREE

Rotisserie Chicken, Baby Kale, Fennel, *and* Green Apple Salad

MAKES 3 SERVINGS

PREP TIME:
15 minutes

—

COOK TIME:
15 minutes

—

One of the greatest convenience items of all time is the supermarket roasted chicken! After shredding the chicken, you should have about 9 ounces of meat, which is perfect for three salads. To lessen the amount of calories and saturated fat, be sure to remove the skin.

1 teaspoon olive oil

1 teaspoon chopped garlic

⅔ cup quinoa

1⅓ cups water

1 cooked rotisserie chicken, meat removed and shredded (about 9 ounces)

1 fennel bulb, core and fronds removed, thinly sliced (about 2 cups)

1 small green apple, julienned (about 1½ cups)

8 tablespoons Honey-Lemon Vinaigrette (page 178), divided

1 (5-ounce) package baby kale

6 tablespoons walnut pieces

1. Heat the oil over medium heat in a saucepan. Once the oil is shimmering, add the garlic and cook for 1 minute, stirring often so that it doesn't burn.

2. Add the quinoa and stir a few times. Add the water and turn the heat up to high. Once the water is boiling, cover the pan and turn the heat down to low. Simmer the quinoa for 15 minutes, or until the water is absorbed. Cool.

3. Place the chicken, fennel, apple, and cooled quinoa in a large bowl. Add 2 tablespoons of the vinaigrette to the bowl and mix to combine.

4. Divide the baby kale, chicken mixture, and walnuts among 3 containers. Pour 2 tablespoons of the remaining vinaigrette into each of 3 sauce containers.

STORAGE *Store covered containers in the refrigerator for up to 5 days.*

TIP *To avoid chopping walnuts, buy walnut pieces instead of walnut halves.*

Per Serving: Total calories: 629; Total fat: 39g; Saturated fat: 6g; Sodium: 727mg; Carbohydrates: 49g; Fiber: 8g; Protein: 29g

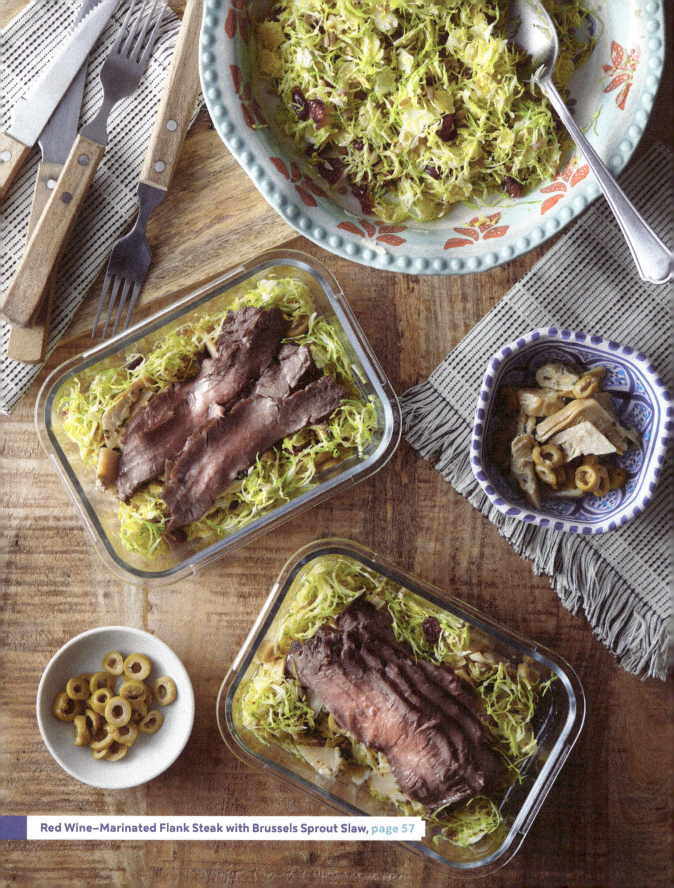

Red Wine–Marinated Flank Steak with Brussels Sprout Slaw, **page 57**

CHAPTER 5

Prep 3

You're pretty much a meal prep pro now, so it's time to add a snack recipe. There's red wine incorporated into two of these dishes, but don't worry—you'll have enough left over to drink! Since there's an extra recipe in this prep, you'll appreciate the fact that one of the entrées is made extra simple with the introduction of the bento-box concept with ingredients that need minimal cooking, if any. With this type of meal, it's useful to follow a formula to create a variety of boxes. Add protein, veggies, whole-grain flatbread or crackers, nuts or seeds, and a dip. You can even add a side of fresh fruit if you like. Before you begin this prep, please note that the steak for the **Red Wine–Marinated Flank Steak** (page 57) needs to marinate for 8 to 24 hours. It's best to do this step the night before you begin the rest of the prep.

Shopping List

PANTRY

- ☐ Artichoke hearts, marinated, 1 (6-ounce) jar
- ☐ Cocoa powder, unsweetened (2 tablespoons)
- ☐ Dried Italian herbs
- ☐ Extra-virgin olive oil
- ☐ Garlic powder
- ☐ Green olives (9)
- ☐ Ground cardamom
- ☐ Ground cinnamon
- ☐ Kosher salt
- ☐ Nutritional yeast (1 bag)
- ☐ Pure maple syrup
- ☐ Soy sauce, low-sodium (1 small bottle)
- ☐ Tomato paste (1 tube)
- ☐ Tomatoes, crushed, no-salt-added, 1 (28-ounce) can

FRESH PRODUCE

- ☐ Banana, ripe (1)
- ☐ Basil, fresh (1 small bunch)
- ☐ Brussels sprouts (12 ounces)
- ☐ Carrots (2 medium)
- ☐ Cucumbers, 4 (6-inch) Persian or 2 (small) English
- ☐ Dill, fresh (1 small bunch)
- ☐ Garlic, chopped (1 jar) or head (1)
- ☐ Lemons (2)
- ☐ Mushrooms, button or cremini (8 ounces)
- ☐ Onion, yellow (1 small)
- ☐ Sugar snap peas (2 cups)

PROTEIN

- ☐ Flank steak (8 ounces)
- ☐ Smoked salmon (8 ounces)

DAIRY

- ☐ Milk, low-fat (2%) (2½ cups)
- ☐ Ricotta cheese, whole-milk, 1 (16-ounce) container

GRAINS, NUTS, SEEDS, AND LEGUMES

- ☐ Almond butter, plain, unsalted, creamy (1 jar)
- ☐ Almond meal (¼ cup)
- ☐ Brown lentils (1-pound bag)
- ☐ Chia seeds (½ cup)
- ☐ Flaxseed, ground (3 tablespoons)
- ☐ Oats, rolled (½ cup)
- ☐ Penne, whole-wheat (1-pound box)
- ☐ Pitas, whole-wheat (4)
- ☐ Sunflower seeds (3 tablespoons)

OTHER

- ☐ Blueberries, frozen, 1 (16-ounce) bag
- ☐ Cranberries, dried (2 tablespoons)
- ☐ Dry red wine, such as red zinfandel, merlot, or cabernet (1 bottle)

Equipment

- ☐ Chef's knife
- ☐ Cutting board
- ☐ Measuring cups and spoons
- ☐ Mixing bowls
- ☐ Spatulas
- ☐ 18-by-13-inch sheet pan
- ☐ Saucepan
- ☐ Soup pot
- ☐ Aluminum foil
- ☐ Resealable gallon-size plastic bag for marinating

Day	Breakfast	Lunch	Dinner	Snack
1	Maple-Cardamom Chia Pudding with Blueberries	Smoked Salmon and Lemon-Dill Ricotta Bento Box	Whole-Wheat Pasta with Lentil Bolognese	Cocoa-Almond Bliss Bites
2	Maple-Cardamom Chia Pudding with Blueberries	Smoked Salmon and Lemon-Dill Ricotta Bento Box	Whole-Wheat Pasta with Lentil Bolognese	Cocoa-Almond Bliss Bites
3	Maple-Cardamom Chia Pudding with Blueberries	Smoked Salmon and Lemon-Dill Ricotta Bento Box	Red Wine–Marinated Flank Steak with Brussels Sprout Slaw	Cocoa-Almond Bliss Bites
4	Maple-Cardamom Chia Pudding with Blueberries	Smoked Salmon and Lemon-Dill Ricotta Bento Box	Whole-Wheat Pasta with Lentil Bolognese	Cocoa-Almond Bliss Bites
5	Maple-Cardamom Chia Pudding with Blueberries	Red Wine–Marinated Flank Steak with Brussels Sprout Slaw	Whole-Wheat Pasta with Lentil Bolognese	Cocoa-Almond Bliss Bites

Step-by-Step Prep

1. Prepare the **Lentil Bolognese** sauce (page 53). While the sauce is simmering, cook the pasta. Once both items are cool, place 1 cup of cooked pasta and 1¼ cups of sauce in each of 4 containers. You will have extra sauce, which can be frozen for a later meal.

2. While the pasta and sauce are cooking, make the **Cocoa-Almond Bliss Bites** (page 55) and place them in the freezer to harden.

3. Make the **Maple-Cardamom Chia Pudding with Blueberries** (page 56), spoon ½ cup into each of 5 containers, and top each container with ½ cup of frozen blueberries. Refrigerate.

4. Preheat the oven to the high broiler setting and cover a sheet pan with foil. Prepare the Brussels sprout slaw from the **Red Wine–Marinated Flank Steak with Brussels Sprout Slaw** recipe (page 57).

5. Remove the **Red Wine–Marinated Flank Steak** (page 57) from the marinade. Broil the steak. While the steak is broiling, start working on the **Artichoke-Olive Compote** (page 173).

6. When the steak is cooked, allow it to rest for 5 to 10 minutes before slicing. Place 1 cup of Brussels sprout slaw in each of 2 containers with ⅓ cup of **Artichoke-Olive Compote** (page 173) beside the sprouts. Because the steak will be reheated, place that in 2 separate containers. Alternatively, if you wish to eat the steak at room temperature, place all 3 items in the same container. After packaging, refrigerate the containers.

7. Prepare the lemon-dill ricotta for the **Smoked Salmon and Lemon-Dill Ricotta Bento Box** recipe (page 59) and place ⅓ cup of the ricotta mixture in each of 4 small containers. Place all the other ingredients in 4 separate containers. Refrigerate the bento boxes and ricotta. Package the pita bread pieces in their own resealable bag and store at room temperature so that they don't get soggy. You will have extra snap peas if you bought a 12-ounce package. Incorporate those as snacks during the week.

8. Remove the **Cocoa-Almond Bliss Bites** (page 55) from the freezer and package 2 bites in each of 5 small containers or small resealable bags. Refrigerate.

Whole-Wheat Pasta *with* Lentil Bolognese

PREP TIME:
15 minutes

———

COOK TIME:
55 minutes

———

Lentils are packed with fiber, protein, and iron. The vitamin C in the tomatoes will actually help increase the absorbability of the iron contained in the lentils. Feel free to substitute a different pasta shape—there is no wrong pasta.

2 tablespoons olive oil, divided

1 small yellow onion, chopped (about 2 cups)

1 tablespoon chopped garlic

2 medium carrots, peeled, halved vertically, and sliced (about 1¼ cup)

8 ounces button or cremini mushrooms, roughly chopped (about 4 cups)

1 teaspoon dried Italian herbs

2 tablespoons tomato paste

½ cup dry red wine

1 (28-ounce) can no-salt-added crushed tomatoes

2 cups water

1 cup uncooked brown lentils

½ teaspoon kosher salt

8 ounces dry whole-wheat penne pasta

¼ cup nutritional yeast

1. Heat a soup pot on medium-high heat with 1 tablespoon of oil. Once the oil is shimmering, add the onion and garlic, and cook for 2 minutes.

2. Add the carrots and mushrooms, then stir and cook for another 5 minutes.

3. Add the Italian herbs and tomato paste, stir to evenly incorporate, and cook for 5 more minutes, without stirring.

4. Add the wine and scrape up any bits from the bottom of the pan. Cook for 2 more minutes.

5. Add the tomatoes, water, lentils, and salt. Bring to a boil, then turn the heat down to low and simmer for 40 minutes.

Continued »

Whole-Wheat Pasta with Lentil Bolognese *continued*

6. While the sauce is cooking, cook the pasta according to the package directions, drain, and cool.

7. When the sauce is done simmering, stir in the remaining 1 tablespoon of oil and the nutritional yeast. Cool the sauce.

8. Combine 1 cup of cooked pasta and 1⅓ cups of sauce in each of 4 containers. Freeze the remaining sauce for a later meal.

STORAGE *Store covered containers in the refrigerator for up to 5 days.*

TIP *Nutritional yeast gives items a hint of savory, nutty, and almost cheese-like flavor. You can find it in the baking aisle, the health-food aisle, or the bulk bins. Two well-known brands are Trader Joe's and Bob's Red Mill.*

Per Serving: Total calories: 570; Total fat: 9g; Saturated fat: 1g; Sodium: 435mg; Carbohydrates: 96g; Fiber: 17g; Protein: 27g

Cocoa-Almond Bliss Bites

**MAKES
10 BITES**

PREP TIME:
10 minutes

———

FREEZE TIME:
1 hour

———

Don't be fooled by the small size of these snacks! The healthy fats and fiber from the almonds and flaxseed make them filling. Sweet but not too sweet, they hit the spot as a snack or even a dessert.

1 medium ripe banana, mashed

3 tablespoons ground flaxseed

½ cup rolled oats

½ cup plain, unsalted almond butter

2 tablespoons unsweetened cocoa powder

¼ cup almond meal

¼ teaspoon ground cinnamon

2 teaspoons pure maple syrup

1. Combine all the ingredients in a medium mixing bowl.
2. Roll the mixture into 10 balls, slightly smaller than a golf ball, and place on a plate.
3. Freeze the bites for 1 hour to harden.
4. Place 2 bites in each of 5 small containers or resealable bags and store in the refrigerator.

STORAGE *Store covered containers or resealable bags in the refrigerator for up to 5 days. If you want to make a big batch, the bites can be frozen for up to 3 months.*

TIP *Almond meal is simply finely ground almonds that resemble the texture of flour. You can find it in the baking aisle of your supermarket where the alternative flours are. Store open bags in the freezer to keep them fresh.*

Per Serving (2 bites): Total calories: 130; Total fat: 9g; Saturated fat: 1g; Sodium: 1mg; Carbohydrates: 11g; Fiber: 3g; Protein: 5g

Maple-Cardamom Chia Pudding *with* Blueberries

MAKES 5 SERVINGS

PREP TIME: 5 minutes

—

Chia seeds are nutritional powerhouses. They are rich in protein, omega-3s, fiber, and antioxidants. To make this recipe vegan, use an unsweetened plant-based beverage, such as almond or cashew milk. If you're looking for a heartier breakfast, add some chopped unsalted pistachios.

2½ cups low-fat (2%) milk

½ cup chia seeds

1 tablespoon plus 1 teaspoon pure maple syrup

¼ teaspoon ground cardamom

2½ cups frozen blueberries

1. Place the milk, chia seeds, maple syrup, and cardamom in a large bowl and stir to combine.

2. Spoon ½ cup of the mixture into each of 5 containers.

3. Place ½ cup of frozen blueberries in each container and stir to combine. Let the pudding sit for at least an hour in the refrigerator before eating.

STORAGE *Store covered containers in the refrigerator for up to 5 days.*

TIP *Please don't buy syrup labeled pancake syrup. It's not real maple syrup and is full of chemicals and artificial ingredients. If your store sells Grade A and Grade B maple syrup, go for the Grade B, because it's less expensive.*

Per Serving: Total calories: 218; Total fat: 8g; Saturated fat: 2g; Sodium: 74mg; Carbohydrates: 28g; Fiber: 10g; Protein: 10g

Red Wine–Marinated Flank Steak
with Brussels Sprout Slaw

PREP TIME:
5 minutes,
plus 8 hours
to marinate

——

COOK TIME:
10 minutes

——

Red wine imparts lots of flavor to meats when used as a marinade. It's best to marinate the meat for at least 8 hours, but up to 24 hours will also yield a delicious result. A dry zinfandel, cabernet sauvignon, merlot, or Syrah is a good wine option. You don't need to use an expensive wine, but you should use one that you want to drink, because you'll have plenty left over.

FOR THE STEAK

8 ounces flank steak, trimmed of visible fat

½ cup red wine

2 tablespoons low-sodium soy sauce

1 tablespoon olive oil

½ teaspoon garlic powder

FOR THE BRUSSELS SPROUT SLAW

8 ounces Brussels sprouts, stemmed, halved, and very thinly sliced

3 tablespoons unsalted sunflower seeds

3 tablespoons freshly squeezed lemon juice

1 tablespoon plus 1 teaspoon olive oil

2 tablespoons dried cranberries

⅛ teaspoon kosher salt

⅔ cup Artichoke-Olive Compote (page 173)

TO MAKE THE STEAK

1. Place all the ingredients for the steak in a gallon-size resealable bag. Allow the steak to marinate overnight or up to 24 hours.

2. Place the oven rack about 6 inches from the heating element. Preheat the oven to the broil setting (use the high setting if you have multiple settings).

Continued »

Red Wine–Marinated Flank Steak
with Brussels Sprout Slaw *continued*

3. Cover a sheet pan with foil. Lift the steak out of the marinade and place on top of the foil-lined sheet pan. Place the pan in the oven and cook for 4 to 6 minutes on one side. Flip the steak over to the other side and broil for 4 to 6 minutes more.

4. Remove from the oven and allow to rest for 5 to 10 minutes. Medium-rare will be about 135°F when an instant-read meat thermometer is inserted.

5. On a cutting board, slice the steak thinly against the grain and divide the steak between 2 containers.

TO MAKE THE BRUSSELS SPROUT SLAW

6. Combine the Brussels sprouts, sunflower seeds, lemon juice, olive oil, cranberries, and salt in a medium bowl.

7. Place 1 cup of Brussels sprout slaw and ⅓ cup of artichoke-olive compote in each of 2 containers. The slaw and compote are meant to be eaten at room temperature, while the steak can be eaten warm. However, if you want to eat the steak at room temperature as well, all the items can be put in the same container.

STORAGE *Store covered containers in the refrigerator for up to 5 days.*

TIP *Alternatively, you can grill the steak on an outdoor grill or indoor grill pan rather than broiling.*

Per Serving: Total calories: 601; Total fat: 31g; Saturated fat: 3g; Sodium: 1,098mg; Carbohydrates: 26g; Fiber: 5g; Protein: 29g

Smoked Salmon *and* Lemon-Dill Ricotta Bento Box

PREP TIME:
10 minutes

——

I love a meal that involves very little chopping and no cooking! This meal is super simple and packed full of nutrients like omega-3s, fiber, protein, calcium, iron, and B$_{12}$. If you are on a low-sodium diet, use roasted salmon instead of smoked salmon.

FOR THE LEMON-DILL RICOTTA

1 (16-ounce) container whole-milk ricotta cheese

1 teaspoon finely grated lemon zest

3 tablespoons chopped fresh dill

FOR THE BENTO BOX

8 ounces smoked salmon

4 (6-inch) Persian cucumbers or 2 small European cucumbers, sliced

2 cups sugar snap peas

4 whole-wheat pitas, each cut into 4 pieces

1. Mix all the ingredients for the lemon-dill ricotta in a medium bowl.
2. Divide the salmon, cucumbers, and snap peas among 4 containers.
3. Place 1 pita in each of 4 resealable bags.
4. Place ½ cup of ricotta spread in each of 4 separate small containers, since it may release some liquid after a couple of days.

STORAGE *Store covered containers in the refrigerator for up to 4 days. Store the pita at room temperature or in the refrigerator.*

TIP *Because you're not using a whole package of pita in this recipe, you can freeze the leftovers if you wish.*

Per Serving: Total calories: 469; Total fat: 20g; Saturated fat: 11g; Sodium: 1,388mg; Carbohydrates: 40g; Fiber: 8g; Protein: 32g

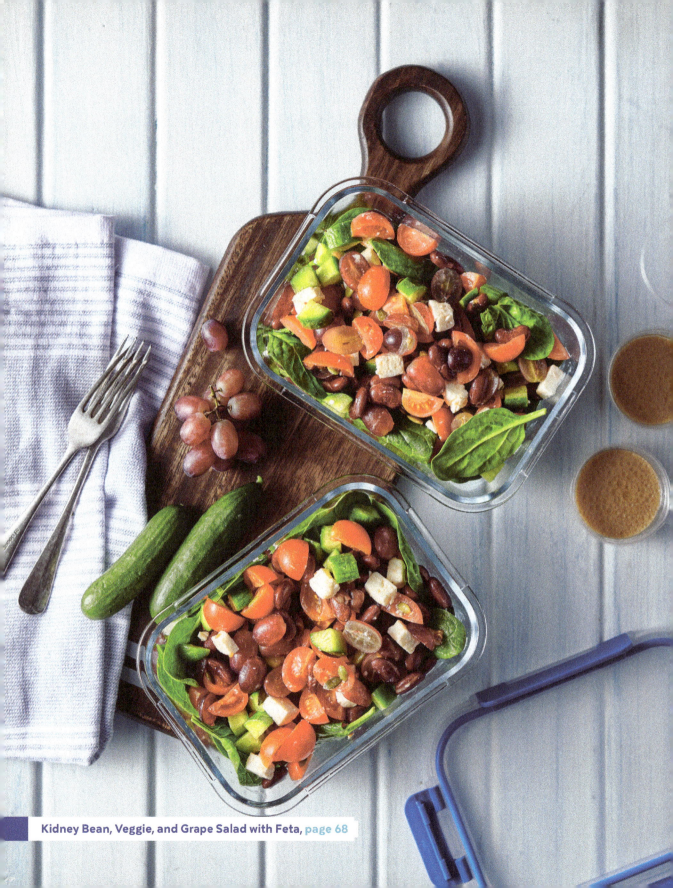

Kidney Bean, Veggie, and Grape Salad with Feta, page 68

CHAPTER 6

Prep 4

This week's prep consists of five recipes for breakfast, lunch, dinner, and a snack. This prep focuses on one-bowl, one-pot recipes and a sheet-pan meal to help you minimize the number of bowls, pots, and pans used. You'll get extra servings from the **Apple, Cinnamon, and Walnut Baked Oatmeal** (page 67) that you can freeze for a later time. This week also incorporates more fruit, including apples at breakfast, grapes in a salad, golden raisins with fish, and strawberries with the snack. Fruit is packed with important vitamins, minerals, antioxidants, and fiber and is a key component of the Mediterranean lifestyle.

Shopping List

PANTRY

☐ Baking powder
☐ Capers (1 jar)
☐ Chicken broth, low-sodium (8 fluid ounces)
☐ Dijon mustard (1 jar)
☐ Dried oregano
☐ Dried thyme leaves
☐ Extra-virgin olive oil
☐ Ground cinnamon
☐ Kosher salt
☐ Pure maple syrup (⅓ cup)
☐ Red wine vinegar (1 bottle)
☐ Smoked paprika
☐ Tomatoes, diced, no-salt-added, 1 (14.5-ounce) can

FRESH PRODUCE

☐ Baby red potatoes (10 ounces)
☐ Baby spinach, 1 (5-ounce) container
☐ Basil, fresh, 1 (½-ounce) package
☐ Cherry tomatoes (10 ounces)
☐ Cucumbers, 4 (6-inch) Persian or 2 (small) English
☐ Garlic, chopped (1 jar) or head (1)
☐ Green apples (3 small, about 1 pound)
☐ Green bell pepper (1 large)
☐ Lemon (1)
☐ Onions, yellow (2 small)
☐ Red bell pepper (1 large)
☐ Red grapes (1½ cups)
☐ Strawberries, fresh (16 ounces)
☐ Zucchini (1 medium)

PROTEIN

☐ Eggs (2)
☐ Chicken sausage, cooked, 1 (12-ounce) package
☐ Shrimp, uncooked, peeled, deveined, medium (6 ounces)
☐ Tilapia or other thin white fish, such as red snapper (8 ounces)

DAIRY

☐ Cottage cheese, low-fat, 1 (16-ounce) container
☐ Feta cheese (½ cup)
☐ Milk, low-fat (2%) (1½ cups)

GRAINS, NUTS, SEEDS, AND LEGUMES

☐ Brown rice, quick-cooking or instant (½ cup)
☐ Dark red kidney beans, low-sodium, 1 (15-ounce) can
☐ Flaxseed, ground (3 tablespoons)
☐ Green pumpkin seeds (pepitas) (½ cup)
☐ Oats, rolled (3 cups)
☐ Pistachios, unsalted (⅔ cup)
☐ Walnut pieces (½ cup)

OTHER

☐ Golden raisins (¼ cup)

Equipment

- ☐ Chef's knife
- ☐ Cutting board
- ☐ Measuring cups and spoons
- ☐ Mixing bowls
- ☐ Spatulas
- ☐ Whisk
- ☐ 8-by-11-inch glass or ceramic baking dish

- ☐ 18-by-13-inch sheet pan
- ☐ Silicone baking mat or parchment paper
- ☐ 12-inch skillet
- ☐ Soup pot or Dutch oven

Day	Breakfast	Lunch	Dinner	Snack
1	Apple, Cinnamon, and Walnut Baked Oatmeal	One-Pot Spanish Chicken Sausage and Shrimp with Rice	Mediterranean Baked Tilapia with Roasted Baby Red Potatoes	Strawberries with Cottage Cheese and Pistachios
2	Apple, Cinnamon, and Walnut Baked Oatmeal	Kidney Bean, Veggie, and Grape Salad with Feta	One-Pot Spanish Chicken Sausage and Shrimp with Rice	Strawberries with Cottage Cheese and Pistachios
3	Apple, Cinnamon, and Walnut Baked Oatmeal	Kidney Bean, Veggie, and Grape Salad with Feta	Mediterranean Baked Tilapia with Roasted Baby Red Potatoes	Strawberries with Cottage Cheese and Pistachios
4	Apple, Cinnamon, and Walnut Baked Oatmeal	One-Pot Spanish Chicken Sausage and Shrimp with Rice	Kidney Bean, Veggie, and Grape Salad with Feta	Strawberries with Cottage Cheese and Pistachios
5	Apple, Cinnamon, and Walnut Baked Oatmeal	Kidney Bean, Veggie, and Grape Salad with Feta	One-Pot Spanish Chicken Sausage and Shrimp with Rice	Strawberries with Cottage Cheese and Pistachios

Step-by-Step Prep

1. Preheat the oven to 350°F. Prepare the **One-Pot Spanish Chicken Sausage and Shrimp with Rice** (page 65). Once you cover it and bring it to a simmer, make the **Apple, Cinnamon, and Walnut Baked Oatmeal** (page 67) and bake it in the oven for 40 minutes.

2. Make the **Kidney Bean, Veggie, and Grape Salad with Feta** (page 68) and the **Dijon Red Wine Vinaigrette** (page 177). Portion out 2 cups of salad and 1 cup of spinach leaves into each of 4 containers and 2 tablespoons of vinaigrette into each of 4 sauce containers. Refrigerate.

3. Chop the ingredients for the **Mediterranean Baked Tilapia with Roasted Baby Red Potatoes** (page 69) and start sautéing the onions and peppers.

4. When the **One-Pot Spanish Chicken Sausage and Shrimp with Rice** (page 65) and the **Apple, Cinnamon, and Walnut Baked Oatmeal** (page 67) are done cooking, allow them to cool and increase the oven temperature to 450°F. Once the food is cooled, place 2 cups of the sausage-and-rice mixture in each of 4 containers. Cut the oatmeal into 8 pieces and place 1 piece in each of 5 containers. Refrigerate. Freeze the other 3 pieces for a later time.

5. Finish the preparation for the onion-and-pepper mixture. Place the potatoes for the **Mediterranean Baked Tilapia** (page 69) in the oven and roast for 10 minutes. While the potatoes are roasting, place the **Strawberries with Cottage Cheese and Pistachios** (page 71) in each of 5 containers and refrigerate.

6. Once the 10-minute timer on the potatoes goes off, place the fish-and-onion mixture on the other half of the pan per the recipe instructions and continue cooking for 10 minutes.

7. When the fish and potatoes are cooked, cool before packing into containers. Once they are cooled, place 1 piece of fish plus half of the veggies and half of the potatoes in each of 2 containers and refrigerate.

One-Pot Spanish Chicken Sausage _and_ Shrimp _with_ Rice

MAKES 4 SERVINGS

PREP TIME:
15 minutes

———

COOK TIME:
30 minutes

———

One-pot meals are awesome! You can cook your protein, whole grain, and veggies all in one shot. Be sure to buy brown rice that's labeled "instant" or "quick cooking." This just means that the rice was partially precooked, then dehydrated. Don't worry, it's still a whole grain!

4 teaspoons olive oil, divided

1 (12-ounce) package cooked chicken sausage, sliced

6 ounces uncooked peeled, deveined medium shrimp

1 large green bell pepper, chopped (about 1½ cups)

1 small yellow onion, chopped (about 2 cups)

2 teaspoons chopped garlic

2 teaspoons smoked paprika

1 teaspoon dried thyme leaves

1 teaspoon dried oregano

½ teaspoon kosher salt

½ cup quick-cooking or instant brown rice

1 (14.5-ounce) can no-salt-added diced tomatoes in juice

1 cup low-sodium chicken broth

1 medium zucchini, halved vertically and sliced into half-moons

1. Heat 2 teaspoons of oil in a soup pot over medium-high heat. When the oil is shimmering, add the sausage and brown for 5 minutes. Add the shrimp and cook for 1 more minute. Remove the sausage and shrimp, and place them on a plate.

2. Add the remaining 2 teaspoons of oil to the pot, and when the oil is shimmering, add the bell pepper, onion, and garlic. Sauté until soft, about 5 minutes.

Continued »

One-Pot Spanish Chicken Sausage and Shrimp with Rice *continued*

3. Add the sausage, shrimp, paprika, thyme, oregano, salt, rice, tomatoes, and broth to the pot, and stir to combine. Bring to a boil, then cover the pot and turn the heat down to low. Simmer for 15 minutes.

4. After 15 minutes, add the zucchini, return the cover to the pot, and continue to simmer for 5 to 10 more minutes, until the zucchini is crisp-tender and the rice has absorbed most of the liquid.

5. Place about 2 cups of the rice mixture in each of 4 containers.

STORAGE *Store covered containers in the refrigerator for up to 5 days.*

TIP *There are many good-quality chicken sausages on the market. Be sure to read the ingredient list to find sausage with simple, whole ingredients, such as chicken, fruit, veggies, beans, and even whole grains.*

Per Serving: Total calories: 333; Total fat: 14g; Saturated fat: 3g; Sodium: 954mg; Carbohydrates: 29g; Fiber: 6g; Protein: 26g

Apple, Cinnamon, *and* Walnut Baked Oatmeal

MAKES 8 SERVINGS

PREP TIME:
10 minutes

____

COOK TIME:
40 minutes

____

When making this recipe, don't peel the apples! The skin adds flavor, texture, and fiber. This recipe calls for low-fat milk, but feel free to use any unsweetened plant-based beverage instead.

Cooking spray or oil for greasing the pan

3 small Granny Smith apples (about 1 pound), skin-on, chopped into ½-inch dice

3 cups rolled oats

1 teaspoon baking powder

3 tablespoons ground flaxseed

1 teaspoon ground cinnamon

2 eggs

¼ cup olive oil

1½ cups low-fat (2%) milk

⅓ cup pure maple syrup

½ cup walnut pieces (if you buy walnut halves, roughly chop the nuts)

1. Preheat the oven to 350°F and spray an 8-by-11-inch baking dish with cooking spray or rub with oil.

2. Combine the apples, oats, baking powder, flaxseed, cinnamon, eggs, oil, milk, and maple syrup in a large mixing bowl and pour into the prepared baking dish.

3. Sprinkle the walnut pieces evenly across the oatmeal and bake for 40 minutes.

4. Allow the oatmeal to cool and cut it into 8 pieces. Place 1 piece in each of 5 containers. Take the other 3 pieces and either eat as a snack during the week or freeze for a later time.

STORAGE *Store covered containers in the refrigerator for up to 6 days. If frozen, oatmeal will last 6 months.*

TIP *For you to absorb the nutrients in the flaxseed, the seeds must be ground. Grind whole seeds in a spice grinder or buy ground flaxseed.*

Per Serving: Total calories: 349; Total fat: 18g; Saturated fat: 3g; Sodium: 108mg; Carbohydrates: 43g; Fiber: 6g; Protein: 9g

Kidney Bean, Veggie, *and* Grape Salad *with* Feta

MAKES 4 SERVINGS

PREP TIME:
15 minutes
—

Sometimes a big salad with tons of veggies just hits the spot. You'll never feel too tired to go back to work after having a fiber-rich and fresh meal like this. You can use any type of bean, and feel free to mix up the veggies if you have other types on hand.

1½ cups red grapes, halved

1 (15-ounce) can red kidney beans, drained and rinsed

10 ounces cherry tomatoes, halved (quartered if tomatoes are large)

4 (6-inch) Persian cucumbers, quartered vertically and chopped

½ cup green pumpkin seeds (pepitas)

½ cup feta cheese

2½ ounces baby spinach leaves (about 4 cups)

½ cup Dijon Red Wine Vinaigrette (page 177)

1. Place the grapes, kidney beans, cherry tomatoes, cucumbers, pumpkin seeds, and feta in a large mixing bowl and mix to combine.

2. Place 2 cups of the salad mixture in each of 4 containers. Then place 1 cup of spinach leaves on top of each salad. Pour 2 tablespoons of vinaigrette into each of 4 sauce containers. Refrigerate all the containers.

STORAGE *Store covered containers in the refrigerator for up to 5 days.*

TIP *Because the salad contains items with high moisture content, such as tomatoes and cucumbers, placing the spinach on top of those items, rather than mixing it in, will keep the leaves from getting soggy.*

Per Serving: Total calories: 435; Total fat: 25g; Saturated fat: 6g; Sodium: 435mg; Carbohydrates: 37g; Fiber: 10g; Protein: 16g

Mediterranean Baked Tilapia *with* Roasted Baby Red Potatoes

PREP TIME:
15 minutes

———

COOK TIME:
35 minutes

———

I've been making a version of this dish for years. The combination of salty, sweet, and sour ingredients balances really well. You'll want to package up the potatoes immediately after they cool so you don't snack on them throughout your prep! They're so good!

3 teaspoons olive oil, divided

1 small yellow onion, very thinly sliced (about 2½ cups)

1 large red bell pepper, thinly sliced (about 2 cups)

10 ounces baby red potatoes, quartered (about 1-inch pieces)

⅜ teaspoon kosher salt, divided

1 teaspoon chopped garlic

1 tablespoon capers, drained, rinsed, and roughly chopped

¼ cup golden raisins

1 (½-ounce) pack fresh basil, roughly chopped

2½ ounces baby spinach, large leaves torn in half (about 4 cups)

2 teaspoons freshly squeezed lemon juice

8 ounces tilapia or other thin white fish (see tip on page 70)

1. Preheat the oven to 450°F. Line a sheet pan with a silicone baking mat or parchment paper.

2. Heat 2 teaspoons of oil in a 12-inch skillet over medium heat. When the oil is shimmering, add the onions and peppers. Cook for 12 minutes, stirring occasionally. The onions should be very soft.

3. While the onions and peppers are cooking, place the potatoes on the sheet pan and toss with ⅛ teaspoon of salt and the remaining 1 teaspoon of oil. Spread the potatoes out evenly across half of the pan. Roast in the oven for 10 minutes.

Continued »

Mediterranean Baked Tilapia with Roasted Baby Red Potatoes *continued*

4. Once the onions are soft, add the garlic, capers, raisins, basil, ⅛ teaspoon of salt, and the spinach. Stir to combine and cook for 3 more minutes to wilt the spinach.

5. Carefully remove the sheet pan from the oven after 10 minutes. Add half of the onion mixture to the empty side of the pan to form a nest for the fish. Place the fish on top and season with the remaining ⅛ teaspoon of salt and the lemon juice. Spread the rest of the onion mixture evenly across the top of the fish.

6. Place the pan back in the oven and cook for 10 minutes. The fish should be flaky.

7. When the fish and potatoes have cooled, place 1 piece of fish plus half of the potatoes and half of the onion mixture in each of 2 containers. Refrigerate.

STORAGE *Store covered containers in the refrigerator for up to 4 days.*

TIP *You can use any thin white fish for this dish, such as red snapper, flounder, or sole.*

Per Serving: Total calories: 427; Total fat: 9g; Saturated fat: 2g; Sodium: 952mg; Carbohydrates: 59g; Fiber: 10g; Protein: 31g

Strawberries *with* Cottage Cheese *and* Pistachios

PREP TIME:
5 minutes

———

I adore cottage cheese because it is delicious, filling, and packed with protein, calcium, and vitamin B_{12}. You can swap out the strawberries for any fruit that's in season or looks tasty to you!

16 ounces low-fat cottage cheese

16 ounces strawberries, hulled and sliced

½ cup plus 2 tablespoons unsalted shelled pistachios

1. Spoon ⅓ cup of cottage cheese into each of 5 containers.
2. Top each scoop of cottage cheese with ⅔ cup of strawberries and 2 tablespoons of pistachios.
3. Refrigerate.

STORAGE *Store covered containers in the refrigerator for up to 5 days.*

TIP *Did you know cottage cheese is either "wet" or "dry"? The difference lies in the amount of milk and cream added to the curds, with "wet" being the more traditional variety. A drier cottage cheese also usually contains less sodium. Try out different brands to see what you like best.*

Per Serving: Total calories: 184; Total fat: 9g; Saturated fat: 2g; Sodium: 265mg; Carbohydrates: 14g; Fiber: 4g; Protein: 15g

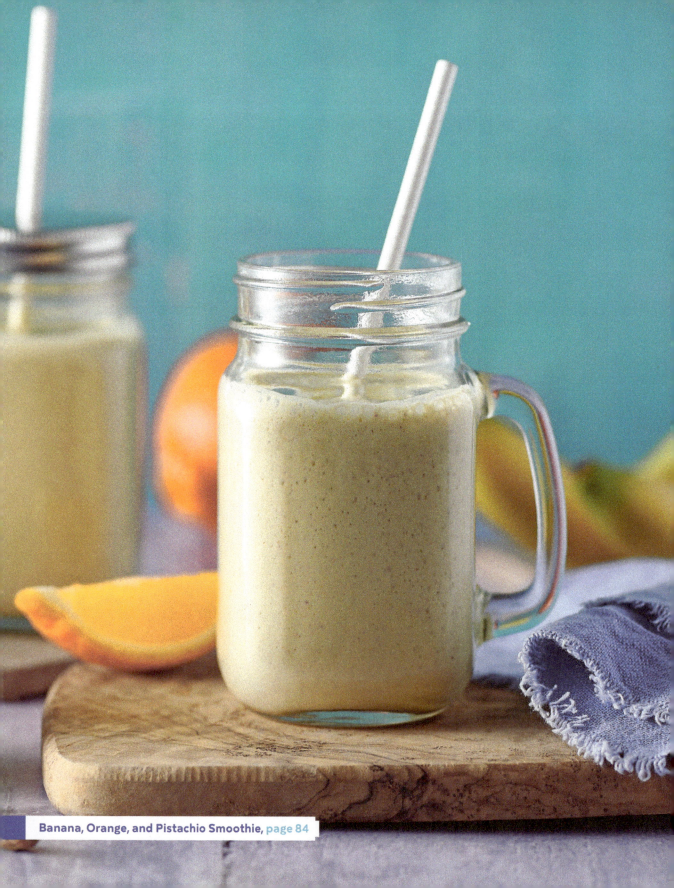

Banana, Orange, and Pistachio Smoothie, **page 84**

CHAPTER 7

Prep 5

We're mixing things up a bit this week by adding a sixth recipe. You'll still get breakfast, lunch, dinner, and a snack, but now there are multiple breakfast options so that you don't have to eat the same thing every morning. The two breakfast options are polar opposites in texture: a smoothie to drink on a couple of days and a crispbread with berry-chia jam and mascarpone for another option. You'll also be using a number of super-flavorful, health-promoting herbs and spices in the entrées this week, including herbes de Provence, fresh dill and basil, cumin, coriander, and caraway seeds.

Shopping List

PANTRY

- ☐ Artichoke hearts, 1 (14-ounce) can
- ☐ Caraway seeds
- ☐ Dijon mustard
- ☐ Extra-virgin olive oil
- ☐ Garlic powder
- ☐ Ground coriander
- ☐ Ground cumin
- ☐ Herbes de Provence
- ☐ Honey
- ☐ Kosher salt
- ☐ Olives, pitted kalamata or niçoise (⅓ cup)
- ☐ Pure maple syrup
- ☐ Red chili flakes
- ☐ Tomato paste

FRESH PRODUCE

- ☐ Basil, fresh, 1 (½-ounce) package
- ☐ Bananas, ripe (3 medium)
- ☐ Cherry tomatoes (10 ounces)
- ☐ Cucumbers, 2 (6-inch) Persian or 1 English
- ☐ Dill, fresh (1 large bunch)
- ☐ Eggplant, 1 (14-ounce)
- ☐ Garlic, chopped (1 jar) or head (1)
- ☐ Kale and cabbage slaw, 1 (11-ounce) bag
- ☐ Lemons (2)
- ☐ Onions, yellow (2 small)
- ☐ Strawberries (1 pint)
- ☐ Zucchini (3 medium)

PROTEIN

- ☐ Chicken, ground lean (½ pound; freeze the other ½ pound if you can only buy a 1-pound pack)
- ☐ Tofu, super-firm (1 pound)
- ☐ Tuna, light, packed in water, 2 (5-ounce) cans

DAIRY

- ☐ Feta cheese, 1 (5-ounce) container
- ☐ Greek yogurt, low-fat (2%), 1 (17.6-ounce) container
- ☐ Mascarpone cheese, 1 (8-ounce) container

GRAINS, NUTS, SEEDS, AND LEGUMES

- ☐ Almonds, whole, unsalted (⅔ cup)
- ☐ Brown lentils (⅓ cup)
- ☐ Brown rice, long-grain (⅓ cup)
- ☐ Chia seeds (2 tablespoons plus 2 teaspoons)
- ☐ Crispbread (1 package)
- ☐ Green pumpkin seeds (pepitas) (½ cup)
- ☐ Pistachios, unsalted, shelled (¾ cup)
- ☐ Popcorn, ready-to-eat, lightly salted, 1 (4.5-ounce) bag

- [ ] Apricot halves, dried (12)
- [ ] Dry white wine, such as sauvignon blanc (1 bottle)
- [ ] Edamame, frozen, 1 package
- [ ] Mixed berries, frozen, 1 (1-pound) bag
- [ ] Orange juice (1½ cups)

Equipment

- [ ] Chef's knife
- [ ] Cutting board
- [ ] Measuring cups and spoons
- [ ] Mixing bowls
- [ ] Spatulas
- [ ] Whisk
- [ ] 18-by-13-inch sheet pan
- [ ] Silicone baking mat or parchment paper
- [ ] 12-inch skillet
- [ ] Saucepan
- [ ] Blender

Day	Breakfast	Lunch	Dinner	Snack
1	Banana, Orange, and Pistachio Smoothie	Tuna, Kale Slaw, Edamame, and Strawberry Salad	Tofu and Vegetable Provençal	Popcorn Trail Mix
2	Crispbread with Mascarpone and Berry-Chia Jam	Tuna, Kale Slaw, Edamame, and Strawberry Salad	Spiced Chicken-Stuffed Zucchini with Brown Rice and Lentils	Banana, Orange, and Pistachio Smoothie
3	Banana, Orange, and Pistachio Smoothie	Tofu and Vegetable Provençal	Spiced Chicken-Stuffed Zucchini with Brown Rice and Lentils	Popcorn Trail Mix
4	Crispbread with Mascarpone and Berry-Chia Jam	Tuna, Kale Slaw, Edamame, and Strawberry Salad	Tofu and Vegetable Provençal	Popcorn Trail Mix
5	Crispbread with Mascarpone and Berry-Chia Jam	Tofu and Vegetable Provençal	Spiced Chicken-Stuffed Zucchini with Brown Rice and Lentils	Popcorn Trail Mix

Step-by-Step Prep

1. Marinate the tofu for **Tofu and Vegetable Provençal** (page 77) for 1 hour.

2. Squeeze the juice from 2 lemons and set aside for easy access. Make the jam for the **Crispbread with Mascarpone and Berry-Chia Jam** (page 79) and place in the refrigerator to thicken for 1 hour.

3. Preheat the oven to 400°F. Prepare the **Brown Rice and Lentils** from the **Spiced Chicken-Stuffed Zucchini** (page 80) recipe. While the rice is cooking, prepare the stuffed zucchini and bake in the oven for 20 minutes. Once the rice and lentils are done, mix in the oil and dill and cool. Once the zucchini is done, set it aside to cool. When everything has cooled, place 2 stuffed zucchini and ⅔ cup of rice and lentils in each of 3 containers and refrigerate. You will have an extra serving of rice and lentils, which you can freeze for a later time.

4. Keep the oven at 400°F. Prepare the vegetable ragout for the **Tofu and Vegetable Provençal** (page 77) and cook for 20 minutes. By this time, the tofu should be done marinating. While the vegetables are cooking, bake the tofu for a total of 30 minutes, flipping the pieces after 15 minutes. Cool everything down, then place 1½ cups of vegetables and ½ cup of tofu in each of 4 containers. Refrigerate.

5. Prepare the **Tuna, Kale Slaw, Edamame, and Strawberry Salad** (page 82) and the **Honey-Lemon Vinaigrette** (page 178). Divide the tuna, followed by the salad, among 3 containers. Place 2 tablespoons of dressing in each of 3 sauce containers.

6. Package the **Crispbread with Mascarpone and Berry-Chia Jam** (page 79) by placing 2 crispbreads in each of 3 resealable sandwich bags. Place 1 tablespoon of mascarpone and 2 tablespoons of jam in each of 3 containers with dividers. Alternatively, put the mascarpone and jam in separate small sauce containers.

7. Make the **Banana, Orange, and Pistachio Smoothie** (page 84) and pour 1¾ cup into each of 3 smoothie cups.

8. Make the **Popcorn Trail Mix** (page 85) and scoop about ⅓ cup of the almond mixture into each of 5 containers or resealable sandwich bags. Place ¾ cup of popcorn in each of 5 separate containers or resealable bags.

Tofu *and* Vegetable Provençal

**MAKES
4 SERVINGS**

PREP TIME:
15 minutes,
plus 1 hour
to marinate

———

COOK TIME:
30 minutes

———

If you think you don't like tofu because of the soft texture, you're buying the wrong tofu! Try buying super-firm (sometimes called "high-protein") tofu, which is even firmer than extra firm. There's no need to drain and press! The texture is similar to paneer, the Indian cheese.

FOR THE TOFU

1 pound super-firm tofu, cut into ¾-inch cubes

2 tablespoons freshly squeezed lemon juice

2 tablespoons olive oil

1 teaspoon garlic powder

1 teaspoon herbes de Provence

¼ teaspoon kosher salt

FOR THE VEGETABLE RAGOUT

4 teaspoons olive oil, divided

1 (14-ounce) eggplant, cubed into 1-inch pieces (5 to 6 cups)

1 small yellow onion, chopped (about 2 cups)

2 teaspoons chopped garlic

10 ounces cherry tomatoes, halved if tomatoes are fairly large

1 (14-ounce) can artichoke hearts, drained

1 teaspoon herbes de Provence

¼ teaspoon kosher salt

½ cup dry white wine, such as sauvignon blanc

⅓ cup pitted kalamata olives, roughly chopped

1 (½-ounce) package fresh basil, chopped

TO MAKE THE TOFU

1. Place the tofu in a container with the lemon juice, oil, garlic powder, herbes de Provence, and salt. Allow to marinate for 1 hour.

2. When you're ready to cook the tofu, preheat the oven to 400°F and line a sheet pan with a silicone baking mat or

Continued »

Tofu and Vegetable Provençal *continued*

parchment paper. Lift the tofu out of the marinade and place it on the sheet pan. Bake for 30 minutes, flipping the tofu over after 15 minutes. Cool, then place about ½ cup of tofu cubes in each of 4 containers.

TO MAKE THE VEGETABLE RAGOUT

3. While the tofu is marinating, heat 2 teaspoons of oil in a 12-inch skillet over medium-high heat. When the oil is shimmering, add the eggplant and cook for 4 minutes, stirring occasionally. Remove the eggplant and place on a plate.

4. Add the remaining 2 teaspoons of oil to the pan, and add the onion and garlic. Cook for 2 minutes. Add the tomatoes and cook for 5 more minutes. Add the eggplant, artichokes, herbes de Provence, salt, and wine. Cover the pan, lower the heat, and simmer for 20 minutes.

5. Turn the heat off and stir in the olives and basil.

6. Spoon about 1½ cups of vegetables into each of the 4 tofu containers.

STORAGE *Store covered containers in the refrigerator for up to 5 days.*

TIP *Herbes de Provence is a mixture of dried savory, fennel, thyme, rosemary, and lavender. Some mixes may include basil, marjoram, tarragon, and parsley. If you wish to prepare your own herbes de Provence, use equal parts thyme, savory, marjoram, and basil to ⅔ rosemary, ⅓ basil, ⅓ tarragon, ⅓ fennel seeds, and just a dash of lavender buds.*

Per Serving: Total calories: 362; Total fat: 17g; Saturated fat: 3g; Sodium: 728mg; Carbohydrates: 32g; Fiber: 9g; Protein: 23g

Crispbread *with* Mascarpone *and* Berry-Chia Jam

MAKES 3 SERVINGS, PLUS AN EXTRA ⅔ CUP OF JAM THAT CAN BE FROZEN

Crispbread is a large, hearty cracker that makes a great vehicle for sweet and savory toppings. While technically Scandinavian, it fits well into a Mediterranean diet. My favorite crispbread is a gluten-free version from Trader Joe's made from a variety of seeds. You can also replace the crispbread with brown rice cakes.

PREP TIME:
10 minutes

____

COOK TIME:
5 minutes, plus 1 hour to firm in the refrigerator

____

1 (1-pound) bag frozen mixed berries

2 teaspoons freshly squeezed lemon juice

2 teaspoons pure maple syrup

2 tablespoons plus 2 teaspoons chia seeds

6 slices crispbread

3 tablespoons mascarpone cheese

1. Place the frozen berries in a saucepan over medium heat. When the berries are defrosted, about 5 minutes, mash with a potato masher. You can leave them chunky.

2. Turn the heat off and add the lemon juice, maple syrup, and chia seeds.

3. Allow the jam to cool, then place in the refrigerator to thicken for about an hour.

4. Place 2 slices of crispbread in each of 3 resealable sandwich bags. Place 1 tablespoon of mascarpone and 2 tablespoons of jam in each of 3 containers with dividers. Alternatively, put the mascarpone and jam in separate small sauce containers.

STORAGE *Store crispbread at room temperature and jam and mascarpone in the refrigerator. Mascarpone will last for 7 days in the refrigerator, while jam will last for 2 weeks. Jam can be frozen for up to 3 months.*

Per Serving: Total calories: 265; Total fat: 9g; Saturated fat: 3g; Sodium: 105mg; Carbohydrates: 40g; Fiber: 14g; Protein: 6g

Spiced Chicken-Stuffed Zucchini *with* Brown Rice *and* Lentils

MAKES 3 SERVINGS

Stuffed vegetables are very popular in many Mediterranean countries, especially in the eastern Mediterranean. Between the stuffed zucchini and the pilaf, this is a hearty meal packed with protein, even though each portion only contains 2⅔ ounces of chicken.

PREP TIME:
15 minutes
—

COOK TIME:
35 minutes
—

FOR THE BROWN RICE AND LENTILS

⅓ **cup long-grain brown rice**

1⅔ **cups water**

⅛ **teaspoon kosher salt**

⅓ **cup brown lentils**

2 **teaspoons olive oil**

3 **tablespoons chopped fresh dill**

FOR THE STUFFED ZUCCHINI

3 **medium zucchini, halved lengthwise and flesh scooped out with a teaspoon (zucchini flesh reserved)**

3 **teaspoons olive oil, divided**

1 **small yellow onion, chopped**

1 **teaspoon chopped garlic**

½ **pound ground lean chicken**

¾ **teaspoon ground cumin**

¾ **teaspoon ground coriander**

¾ **teaspoon caraway seeds**

⅛ **teaspoon red chili flakes**

3 **tablespoons tomato paste**

¼ **teaspoon kosher salt**

¼ **cup feta cheese**

TO MAKE THE BROWN RICE AND LENTILS

1. Place the rice, water, and salt in a saucepan over high heat. Once the water is boiling, cover the pan and reduce the heat to low. Simmer for 15 minutes.

2. After 15 minutes, add the lentils and stir. Cover the pan and cook for another 15 minutes.

3. If there is a little bit of water still in the pan after the rice and lentils are tender, cook uncovered for a couple of minutes.

4. Stir in the oil and chopped dill.

5. Once the mixture has cooled, place ⅔ cup in each of 3 containers.

TO MAKE THE STUFFED ZUCCHINI

6. Preheat the oven to 400°F and line a sheet pan with a silicone baking mat or parchment paper. Place the zucchini boats on a lined sheet pan and coat with 1 teaspoon of oil.

7. In a 12-inch skillet, heat the remaining 2 teaspoons of oil over medium-high heat. When the oil is shimmering, add the onion and garlic and cook for 5 minutes. Add the zucchini flesh and cook for 2 more minutes.

8. Add the ground chicken, breaking it up with a spatula. Cook for 5 more minutes.

9. Add the cumin, coriander, caraway seeds, chili flakes, tomato paste, and salt, and cook for another 2 minutes.

10. Mound the chicken mixture into the zucchini boats. Top each zucchini boat with 2 teaspoons of feta cheese. Bake for 20 minutes.

11. Once cooled, place 2 zucchini halves in each of the 3 rice-and-lentil containers.

STORAGE *Store covered containers in the refrigerator for up to 5 days. Brown rice and lentils can be frozen for up to 3 months.*

TIP *If your supermarket carries it, choose a crumbled creamy French feta. The taste is rich and salty, and it melts better than some of the drier feta options.*

Per Serving: Total calories: 414; Total fat: 19g; Saturated fat: 5g; Sodium: 645mg; Carbohydrates: 39g; Fiber: 10g; Protein: 26g

Tuna, Kale Slaw, Edamame, *and* Strawberry Salad

PREP TIME:
15 minutes

—

Tuna salad doesn't always have to be a mound of tuna and mayo. Try making salads with canned tuna or salmon, piles of veggies, and a citrus vinaigrette. Adding edamame adds protein and texture, while the strawberries add sweetness and vitamin C.

2 (5-ounce) cans light tuna packed in water

8 tablespoons Honey-Lemon Vinaigrette (page 178), divided

3 cups prepackaged kale-and-cabbage slaw

1 cup shelled frozen edamame, thawed

2 Persian cucumbers, quartered vertically and chopped

1¼ cups sliced strawberries

3 tablespoons chopped fresh dill

1. Place the tuna in a small bowl and mix with 2 tablespoons of vinaigrette.

2. In a large mixing bowl, place the slaw, edamame, cucumbers, strawberries, and dill. Toss to combine.

3. Place ⅓ cup of tuna in each of 3 containers. Place one third of the salad on top of the tuna in each container to lessen the chance of the salad getting soggy. Spoon 2 tablespoons of the remaining vinaigrette into each of 3 separate sauce containers.

Store covered containers in the refrigerator for up to 4 days.

If you're not a fan of the texture of canned tuna, which can be mushy sometimes, try the tuna in pouches. The tuna isn't packed with water and comes in firmer chunks. The downside is that it costs more than the canned option.

Per Serving: Total calories: 317; Total fat: 18g; Saturated fat: 2g; Sodium: 414mg; Carbohydrates: 22g; Fiber: 9g; Protein: 22g

Banana, Orange, *and* Pistachio Smoothie

MAKES 3 SERVINGS

PREP TIME:
5 minutes

—

This smoothie comes from my friend Sandra Castro, who is a fantastic cook and baker. She likes to add a touch of honey to the blender if the bananas aren't super ripe. This yogurt-based smoothie, enhanced by nutrient-rich pistachios, packs in a whopping 26 grams of protein!

1 (17.6-ounce) container plain low-fat (2%) Greek yogurt

3 very ripe medium bananas

1½ cups orange juice

¾ cup unsalted shelled pistachios

1. Place all the ingredients in a blender and blend until smooth.
2. Pour 1¾ cups of the smoothie into each of 3 smoothie containers.

STORAGE *Store covered containers in the refrigerator for up to 4 days.*

TIP *Don't throw away super-ripe bananas. Place peeled bananas in the freezer so that you always have some on hand for smoothies.*

Per Serving: Total calories: 469; Total fat: 19g; Saturated fat: 4g; Sodium: 71mg; Carbohydrates: 55g; Fiber: 3g; Protein: 26g

Popcorn Trail Mix

MAKES 5 SERVINGS

PREP TIME:
5 minutes

Trail mix is delicious, but the serving size is always so small! This recipe adds popcorn to add lightness and give you a larger serving size. Plus, popcorn is a whole grain. There are a number of great ready-to-eat popcorn brands in supermarkets, so you don't have to make your own.

12 dried apricot halves, quartered

⅔ cup whole, unsalted almonds

½ cup green pumpkin seeds (pepitas)

4 cups air-popped lightly salted popcorn

1. Place the apricots, almonds, and pumpkin seeds in a medium bowl and toss with clean hands to evenly mix.

2. Scoop about ⅓ cup of the mixture into each of 5 containers or resealable sandwich bags. Place ¾ cup of popcorn in each of 5 separate containers or resealable bags. You will have one extra serving.

3. Mix the popcorn and the almond mixture together when it's time to eat. (The apricots make the popcorn stale quickly, which is why they're stored separately.)

STORAGE *Store covered containers or resealable bags at room temperature for up to 5 days.*

TIP *Rather than individually quartering apricots, speed things up by stacking 4 apricots on top of each other at a time and quartering the stack.*

Per Serving: Total calories: 244; Total fat: 16g; Saturated fat: 2g; Sodium: 48mg; Carbohydrates: 19g; Fiber: 5g; Protein: 10g

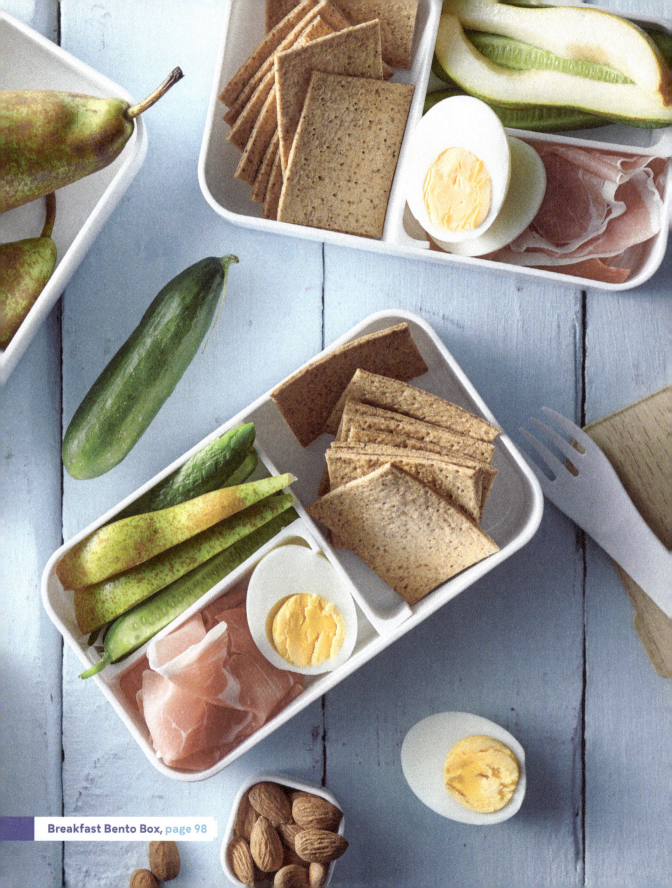

Breakfast Bento Box, page 98

CHAPTER 8

Prep 6

Congratulations on making it to meal prep week 6! I'm sure you've discovered many of your own meal prep tips and tricks over the past five weeks. Breakfast, lunch, dinner, and snacks are included with the six recipes for this week, and you'll find that the **Chocolate–Peanut Butter Yogurt with Berries** (page 99) can actually double as a dessert. Almost all the cooking for this prep will take place on the stovetop. The oven will only be in use for one recipe. This week we're also using some of my favorite cost-effective proteins that give you a big bang for your buck, such as canned salmon, chickpeas, eggs, Greek yogurt, peanut butter, and pork tenderloin. Please note that the **Chutney-Dijon Pork Tenderloin** (page 91) requires at least 8 hours to marinate. Either start this process the night before prep, or if you prep at night, marinate during the morning before your prep time.

Shopping List

PANTRY

- ☐ Capers
- ☐ Cocoa powder, unsweetened
- ☐ Dijon mustard
- ☐ Extra-virgin olive oil
- ☐ Garlic powder
- ☐ Kosher salt
- ☐ Mango or apricot chutney
- ☐ Pure maple syrup
- ☐ Sumac
- ☐ Sun-dried tomatoes
- ☐ Tahini

FRESH PRODUCE

- ☐ Avocado, ripe (1 medium)
- ☐ Baby carrots, 1 (1-pound) bag
- ☐ Belgian endive (2 heads)
- ☐ Berries of your choice, fresh or frozen (1 cup)
- ☐ Cherry tomatoes (10 ounces)
- ☐ Cucumbers, 6 (6-inch Persian) or 1 (large) English
- ☐ Garlic, chopped (1 jar) or head (1)
- ☐ Green beans (1 pound)
- ☐ Kale, lacinato or curly, 1 (7-ounce) bunch
- ☐ Lemons (3)
- ☐ Mint (1 large bunch)
- ☐ Mushrooms (4 ounces; buy sliced, if desired)
- ☐ Parsley (2 bunches)
- ☐ Pear (1 large)
- ☐ Shallot (1 medium)
- ☐ Tarragon (1 bunch)

PROTEIN

- ☐ Eggs (4 large)
- ☐ Pork tenderloin (8 ounces; freeze half if you can only find a 1-pound package)
- ☐ Prosciutto, sliced (2 ounces)
- ☐ Salmon, boneless, skinless, 2 (6-ounce) cans

DAIRY

- ☐ Greek yogurt, low-fat (2%), 1 (16-ounce) container (2 containers if you choose to make the Garlic Yogurt Sauce for the salmon cakes)

GRAINS, NUTS, SEEDS, AND LEGUMES

- ☐ Almonds, whole, unsalted (20)
- ☐ Bulgur wheat (⅔ cup)
- ☐ Chickpeas, low-sodium, 2 (15.5-ounce) cans
- ☐ Crackers, whole-grain (1 box)
- ☐ Farro (⅔ cup)
- ☐ Panko bread crumbs (½ cup)
- ☐ Peanut butter, natural-style, unsalted, smooth or chunky (1 jar)

OTHER

- ☐ Dry red wine, such as red zinfandel, merlot, or cabernet (1 bottle)
- ☐ Vegetable or chicken broth, low-sodium (1¼ cups)

Equipment

- ☐ Chef's knife
- ☐ Cutting board
- ☐ Measuring cups and spoons
- ☐ Mixing bowls
- ☐ Spatulas
- ☐ Whisk
- ☐ 18-by-13-inch sheet pan
- ☐ Silicone baking mat or parchment paper

- ☐ 12-inch skillet
- ☐ Soup pot or Dutch oven
- ☐ Saucepan
- ☐ Blender
- ☐ Resealable gallon-size plastic bag or shallow pan for marinating

Day	Breakfast	Lunch	Dinner	Snack
1	Chocolate–Peanut Butter Yogurt with Berries	Sumac Chickpea Bowl	Salmon Cakes with Steamed Green Bean Gremolata	Avocado Green Goddess Dip with Veggie Dippers
2	Breakfast Bento Box	Chutney-Dijon Pork Tenderloin with Mushroom and Kale Farro Pilaf	Salmon Cakes with Steamed Green Bean Gremolata	Chocolate–Peanut Butter Yogurt with Berries
3	Chocolate–Peanut Butter Yogurt with Berries	Salmon Cakes with Steamed Green Bean Gremolata	Sumac Chickpea Bowl	Avocado Green Goddess Dip with Veggie Dippers
4	Breakfast Bento Box	Sumac Chickpea Bowl	Salmon Cakes with Steamed Green Bean Gremolata	Avocado Green Goddess Dip with Veggie Dippers
5	Chocolate–Peanut Butter Yogurt with Berries	Sumac Chickpea Bowl	Chutney-Dijon Pork Tenderloin with Mushroom and Kale Farro Pilaf	Avocado Green Goddess Dip with Veggie Dippers

Step-by-Step Prep

1. Preheat the oven to 500°F. Prepare the mushroom and kale farro pilaf that goes with the **Chutney-Dijon Pork Tenderloin** (page 91). Roast the **Chutney-Dijon Pork Tenderloin** (page 91) while the pilaf is cooking. When the pork is done, allow it to rest for at least 10 minutes before slicing. Cool the farro when done.

2. Prepare the **Salmon Cakes** (page 93) and cook. Allow the cakes to cool.

3. Slice the **Chutney-Dijon Pork Tenderloin** (page 91) and divide the slices between 2 containers, along with 1 heaping cup of the mushroom and kale farro pilaf for each container.

4. Boil the eggs for the **Breakfast Bento Box** (page 98). Once the heat is turned off for the eggs, cook the sumac chickpeas for the **Sumac Chickpea Bowl** (page 95). Cool once done. When the eggs are done, run them under cold water to cool. Make the bulgur for the chickpea bowl and cool. While the bulgur is cooking, prepare the Israeli salad and tahini sauce. Once all the components are prepared, place 1¼ cups of salad in each of 4 containers. Place ¾ cup of chickpeas and ½ cup of bulgur in each of 4 separate microwaveable containers. Place 1 tablespoon of tahini sauce in each of 4 small sauce containers. Refrigerate.

5. Make the steamed green beans from the **Salmon Cakes with Steamed Green Bean Gremolata** (page 93) recipe and cool. Prepare the optional **Garlic Yogurt Sauce** (page 165) if using. When everything has cooled, place 2 salmon cakes and one quarter of the green beans in each of 4 separate containers. If using, place ¼ cup of the Garlic Yogurt Sauce in each of 4 sauce containers.

6. Prepare the **Avocado Green Goddess Dip with Veggie Dippers** (page 97). Place 4 ounces of carrots and half a head of endive leaves in each of 4 containers. Spoon ¼ cup of dip into each of 4 sauce containers.

7. Assemble the components of the **Breakfast Bento Box** (page 98).

8. Make the **Chocolate–Peanut Butter Yogurt with Berries** (page 99). Spoon ½ cup of yogurt and ¼ cup of berries into each of 4 containers.

Chutney-Dijon Pork Tenderloin *with* Mushroom *and* Kale Farro Pilaf

PREP TIME:
20 minutes,
plus 8 hours
to marinate

——

COOK TIME:
40 minutes

——

Prepared chutney is one of those secret ingredients that can be used in so many dishes. Besides using it as a marinade and glaze for meats, you can use it in vinaigrettes, mixed into yogurt for a sweet-and-savory parfait, spread on sandwiches, or thinned as a dipping sauce.

FOR THE PORK

8 ounces pork tenderloin (freeze half if you can only find a 1-pound package)

⅓ cup prepared mango or apricot chutney, plus 1 tablespoon

2 tablespoons Dijon mustard

1 teaspoon chopped garlic

2 teaspoons olive oil

FOR THE MUSHROOM AND KALE FARRO PILAF

2 teaspoons olive oil

4 ounces mushrooms, sliced

1 small bunch (about 7 ounces) lacinato or curly kale, ribs removed, leaves roughly chopped

½ teaspoon chopped garlic

⅔ cup farro

¼ cup dry red wine, such as red zinfandel, merlot, or cabernet

1¼ cups low-sodium vegetable broth (or chicken broth)

¼ teaspoon kosher salt

TO MAKE THE PORK

1. Remove the tough silver skin from the tenderloin with a sharp knife.

2. In a small bowl, combine ⅓ cup of chutney and the mustard, garlic, and oil.

3. Place the pork in a gallon-size resealable bag or shallow dish and rub the chutney mixture over the pork. Marinate for at least 8 hours.

Continued »

Chutney-Dijon Pork Tenderloin with
Mushroom and Kale Farro Pilaf *continued*

4. When you're ready to cook, preheat the oven to 500°F and line a sheet pan with a silicone baking mat or foil.

5. Remove the pork from the marinade and place it on the sheet pan. Discard the marinade. Place the pork in the oven for 10 minutes. Turn it over, rub the remaining 1 tablespoon of chutney over the top and sides, and roast for another 8 minutes. (Don't worry if extra marinade burns on the baking mat. The pork will be okay.)

6. Let the pork cool for at least 10 minutes and slice.

7. Divide the slices between 2 containers.

TO MAKE THE MUSHROOM AND KALE FARRO PILAF

8. Heat the oil in a soup pot or Dutch oven over medium-high heat. When the oil is shimmering, add the mushrooms and cook for 4 minutes.

9. Add the kale and garlic, stir, and cook for another 5 minutes.

10. Add the farro, stir, and cook for 1 minute. Add the red wine and allow to cook for 1 more minute.

11. Add the broth and salt, increase the heat to high, and bring to a boil. Once it is boiling, turn the heat down to low, cover, and simmer for 30 minutes, until the farro is tender but still has some bite to it.

12. After it has cooled, place 1 heaping cup of pilaf in each of the 2 pork containers. Refrigerate.

STORAGE *Store covered containers in the refrigerator for up to 5 days. Freeze farro pilaf for up to 6 months.*

TIP *You always want to use a very sharp knife to remove silver skin from a piece of meat. Try doing this with a flexible boning knife. If you don't want to do it, you can ask the butcher counter folks to do it for you.*

Per Serving: Total calories: 677; Total fat: 18g; Saturated fat: 3g; Sodium: 1,041mg; Carbohydrates: 76g; Fiber: 10g; Protein: 48g

Salmon Cakes *with* Steamed Green Bean Gremolata

MAKES 4 SERVINGS

PREP TIME:
15 minutes

———

COOK TIME:
6 minutes

———

If you think seafood is too expensive to eat at least twice per week, canned salmon is a great option to get your omega-3 fatty acids. You can throw in whatever chopped veggies you have on hand. Serve with Garlic Yogurt Sauce (page 165), if desired.

FOR THE SALMON CAKES

2 (6-ounce) cans skinless, boneless salmon, drained

½ teaspoon garlic powder

⅓ cup minced shallot

2 tablespoons Dijon mustard

2 eggs

½ cup panko bread crumbs

1 tablespoon capers, chopped

1 cup chopped parsley

⅓ cup chopped sun-dried tomatoes

1 tablespoon freshly squeezed lemon juice

1 tablespoon olive oil

FOR THE GREEN BEANS

Zest of 2 lemons (about 2 tablespoons when zested with a Microplane)

¼ cup minced parsley

1 teaspoon minced garlic

¼ teaspoon kosher salt

1 teaspoon olive oil

1 pound green beans, trimmed

TO MAKE THE SALMON CAKES

1. In a large bowl, place the salmon, garlic, shallot, mustard, eggs, bread crumbs, capers, parsley, tomatoes, and lemon juice. Stir well to combine.

2. Form 8 patties and place them on a plate.

Continued »

**Salmon Cakes with Steamed
Green Bean Gremolata** *continued*

3. Heat the oil in a 12-inch skillet over medium-high heat. Once the oil is hot, add the patties. Cook for 3 minutes on each side, or until each side is browned.

4. Place 2 cooled salmon cakes in each of 4 containers.

TO MAKE THE GREEN BEANS

5. In a small bowl, combine the lemon zest, parsley, garlic, salt, and oil.

6. Bring about ¼ to ½ inch of water to a boil in a soup pot, Dutch oven, or skillet.

7. Once the water is boiling, add the green beans, cover, and set a timer for 3 minutes. The green beans should be crisp-tender.

8. Drain the green beans and transfer to a large bowl. Add the gremolata (lemon zest mixture) and toss to combine.

9. Divide the green beans among the 4 salmon cake containers. If using, place ¼ cup of Garlic Yogurt Sauce in each of 4 sauce containers. Refrigerate.

STORAGE *Store covered containers in the refrigerator for up to 5 days. Uncooked patties can be frozen for 3 to 4 months.*

TIP *If you have any leftover leafy greens in the refrigerator, such as kale, chard, or spinach, you can chop those up and use them instead of the parsley.*

Per Serving: Total calories: 268; Total fat: 9g; Saturated fat: 2g; Sodium: 638mg; Carbohydrates: 21g; Fiber: 6g; Protein: 27g

Sumac Chickpea Bowl

PREP TIME:
15 minutes

———

COOK TIME:
25 minutes

———

Chickpeas and lemony sumac are a match made in heaven. Combine that with a fresh Israeli salad and simple whole-grain bulgur, and you've got one of my favorite plant-based bowl meals. It's full of texture, variety, and flavor!

FOR THE BULGUR

⅔ cup uncooked bulgur

1⅓ cups water

⅛ teaspoon kosher salt

1 teaspoon olive oil

FOR THE CHICKPEAS

2 tablespoons olive oil

2 (15.5-ounce) cans low-sodium chickpeas, drained and rinsed

3 tablespoons sumac

¼ teaspoon kosher salt

FOR THE SALAD

4 Persian cucumbers, quartered lengthwise and chopped (about 2 cups)

10 ounces cherry tomatoes, quartered (halved if you have small tomatoes)

¼ cup chopped fresh mint

1 cup chopped fresh parsley

4 teaspoons olive oil

2 tablespoons plus 2 teaspoons freshly squeezed lemon juice

¼ teaspoon kosher salt

FOR THE TAHINI SAUCE

2 tablespoons unsalted tahini

¼ teaspoon garlic powder

5 tablespoons water

TO MAKE THE BULGUR

1. Place the bulgur, water, and salt in a saucepan, and bring to a boil. Once it boils, cover the pot with a lid and turn off the heat. Let the covered pot stand for 20 minutes. Stir the oil into the cooked bulgur. Cool.

2. Place ½ cup of bulgur in each of 4 microwaveable containers.

Continued »

Sumac Chickpea Bowl *continued*

TO MAKE THE CHICKPEAS

3. Heat the oil in a 12-inch skillet over medium-high heat. Once the oil is shimmering, add the chickpeas, sumac, and salt, and stir to coat. Cook for 2 minutes without stirring. Give the chickpeas a stir and cook for another 2 minutes without stirring. Stir and cook for 2 more minutes.

4. Place ¾ cup of cooled chickpeas in each of the 4 bulgur containers.

TO MAKE THE SALAD

5. Combine all the ingredients for the salad in a medium mixing bowl. Taste for salt and lemon, and add more if you need it.

6. Place 1¼ cup of salad in each of 4 containers. These containers will not be reheated.

TO MAKE THE TAHINI SAUCE

7. Combine the tahini and garlic powder in a small bowl. Whisk in 1 tablespoon of water at a time until all 5 tablespoons have been incorporated and a thin sauce has formed. It will thicken as it sits.

8. Place 1 tablespoon of tahini sauce in each of 4 small sauce containers.

STORAGE *Store covered containers in the refrigerator for up to 5 days. When serving, reheat the bulgur and chickpeas, add them to the salad, and drizzle the tahini sauce over the top.*

TIP *When buying canned chickpeas and beans, be sure to compare the numbers on the nutrition facts label. The organic varieties tend to have lower amounts of salt.*

Per Serving: Total calories: 485; Total fat: 19g; Saturated fat: 2g; Sodium: 361mg; Carbohydrates: 67g; Fiber: 19g; Protein: 16g

Avocado Green Goddess Dip *with* Veggie Dippers

MAKES 4 SERVINGS

PREP TIME:
10 minutes

This creamy and lemony dip is a great way to use up leftover fresh herbs. If you have any that aren't on my ingredient list, such as basil, throw them in and try it out. Endive is an underrated veggie, in my opinion. The leaves are the perfect scoopers for dip!

½ teaspoon chopped garlic

1 cup packed fresh parsley leaves

½ cup fresh mint leaves

¼ cup fresh tarragon leaves

¼ teaspoon plus ⅛ teaspoon kosher salt

¼ cup freshly squeezed lemon juice

¼ cup extra-virgin olive oil

½ cup water

1 medium avocado

1 (1-pound) bag baby carrots

2 heads endive, leaves separated

1. Place the garlic, parsley, mint, tarragon, salt, lemon juice, oil, water, and avocado in a blender and blend until smooth.
2. Place 4 ounces of carrots and half a head of endive leaves in each of 4 containers. Spoon ¼ cup of dip into each of 4 sauce containers.

STORAGE *Store covered containers in the refrigerator for up to 5 days.*

TIP *Any crunchy veggie can be used as a dipper, including celery, radishes, bell pepper slices, sugar snap peas, and jicama.*

Per Serving: Total calories: 301; Total fat: 21g; Saturated fat: 2g; Sodium: 373mg; Carbohydrates: 24g; Fiber: 13g; Protein: 23g

DAIRY-FREE

Breakfast Bento Box

PREP TIME:
5 minutes

—

COOK TIME:
12 minutes

—

Bento-box meals are very quick and easy to throw together. This particular box is great for days when you don't have access to a microwave, as it is eaten at room temperature. It also works well as an on-the-go meal, because a knife and fork aren't necessary.

2 eggs

2 ounces sliced prosciutto

20 small whole-grain crackers

20 whole, unsalted almonds (about ¼ cup)

2 (6-inch) Persian cucumbers, sliced

1 large pear, sliced

1. Place the eggs in a saucepan and cover with water. Bring the water to a boil. As soon as the water starts to boil, place a lid on the pan and turn the heat off. Set a timer for 12 minutes.

2. When the timer goes off, drain the hot water and run cold water over the eggs to cool. Peel the eggs when cool and cut in half.

3. Place 2 egg halves and half of the prosciutto, crackers, almonds, cucumber slices, and pear slices in each of 2 containers.

STORAGE *Store covered containers in the refrigerator for up to 5 days.*

TIP *A sprinkle of Everything but the Bagel seasoning from Trader Joe's, Everything seasoning from Walmart, or Simply Organic's Everything Blend is a tasty addition to hardboiled eggs.*

Per Serving: Total calories: 370; Total fat: 20g; Saturated fat: 5g; Sodium: 941mg; Carbohydrates: 35g; Fiber: 7g; Protein: 16g

Chocolate–Peanut Butter Yogurt *with* Berries

PREP TIME:
5 minutes

———

Packed with protein, calcium, probiotics, healthy fats, and antioxidants, this chocolaty snack can actually double as a healthy dessert. If you don't want to use maple syrup, try adding a ripe mashed banana for sweetness.

2 cups low-fat (2%) plain Greek yogurt

4 tablespoons unsweetened cocoa powder

4 tablespoons natural-style peanut butter

1 tablespoon pure maple syrup

1 cup fresh or frozen berries of your choice

1. In a medium bowl, mix the yogurt, cocoa powder, peanut butter, and maple syrup until well combined.

2. Spoon ½ cup of the yogurt mixture and ¼ cup of berries into each of 4 containers.

STORAGE *Store covered containers in the refrigerator for up to 5 days.*

TIP *When buying peanut butter, opt for the unsalted version. Look at the ingredient list; ideally, the only ingredient listed will be peanuts.*

Per Serving: Total calories: 225; Total fat: 12g; Saturated fat: 4g; Sodium: 130mg; Carbohydrates: 19g; Fiber: 4g; Protein: 16g

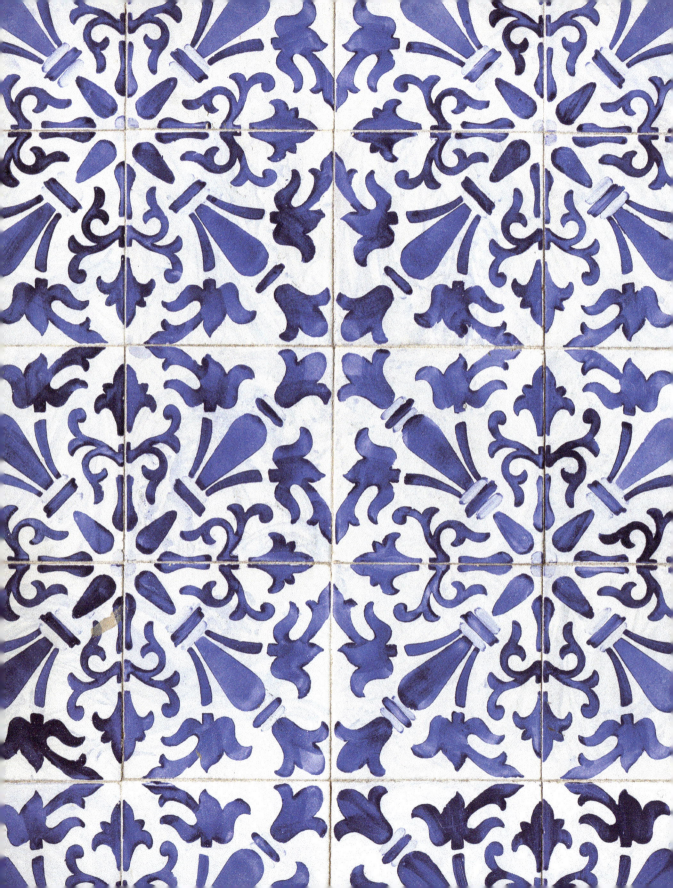

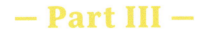

— Part III —

Bonus Meal Prep Recipes

In Part III, you'll find 65 additional recipes beyond the weekly meal preps. Use these recipes as inspiration to create your own custom meal prep menus. This section includes Breakfast; Lunch and Dinner; Dips, Dressings, and Sauces; and Sides, Snacks, and Sweets. Flavors come from all over the Mediterranean, using herbs, spices, and pantry items you should already have on hand from the meal preps. You can also utilize these recipes as springboards for your own creative Mediterranean-style dishes.

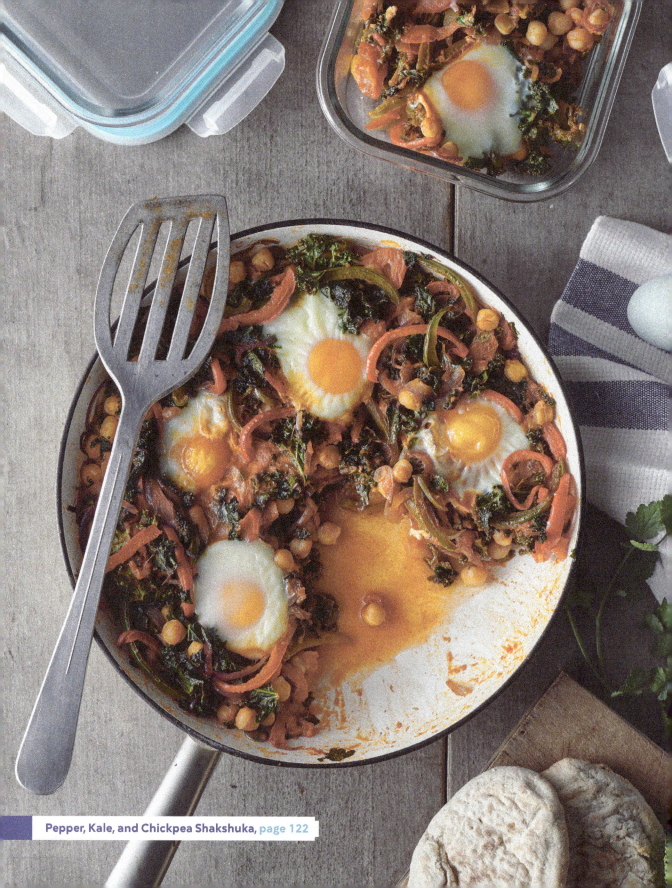

Pepper, Kale, and Chickpea Shakshuka, page 122

Breakfast

Chocolate-Almond Banana Bread

**MAKES
4 SERVINGS**

PREP TIME:
10 minutes

——

COOK TIME:
25 minutes

——

Bananas are always in my freezer for smoothies and banana bread. This grain-free banana bread is cooked in a shallow pan rather than a loaf pan so that it cooks more quickly. The generous serving size is meant for breakfast. If you choose to eat this as a snack, you may want to cut smaller pieces.

Cooking spray or oil to grease the pan

1 cup almond meal

2 large eggs

2 very ripe bananas, mashed

1 tablespoon plus 2 teaspoons maple syrup

½ teaspoon vanilla extract

½ teaspoon baking powder

¼ teaspoon ground cardamom

⅓ cup dark chocolate chips, very roughly chopped

1. Preheat the oven to 350°F and spray an 8-inch cake pan or baking dish with cooking spray or rub with oil.

2. Combine all the ingredients in a large mixing bowl. Then pour the mixture into the prepared pan.

3. Place the pan in the oven and bake for 25 minutes. The edges should be browned, and a paring knife should come out clean when the banana bread is pierced.

4. When cool, slice into 4 wedges and place 1 wedge in each of 4 containers.

STORAGE *Store covered containers at room temperature for up to 2 days, refrigerate for up to 7 days, or freeze for up to 3 months.*

TIP *Almond meal typically contains the almond skins and is slightly coarser than almond flour, which is usually made from blanched almonds. Almond meal is recommended for this recipe, but almond flour can be used interchangeably.*

Per Serving: Total calories: 365; Total fat: 23g; Saturated fat: 6g; Sodium: 105mg; Carbohydrates: 37g; Fiber: 6g; Protein: 10g

Honey, Dried Apricot, *and* Pistachio Yogurt Parfait

Honey, pistachios, and dried apricots are staple ingredients in countries of the eastern Mediterranean. By making your own sweetened yogurt, you get to control the amount of honey used. Taste the yogurt after adding 2 teaspoons of honey. If it's not sweet enough for you, add the remaining 1 teaspoon.

1 (16-ounce) container low-fat (2%) plain Greek yogurt

1 tablespoon honey

½ teaspoon rose water (optional)

½ cup unsalted shelled pistachios, roughly chopped

12 dried apricot halves, quartered

1. Mix the yogurt, honey, and rose water (if using) in a medium bowl.
2. Place ⅔ cup of yogurt in each of 3 containers. Top each mound of yogurt with equal portions of the pistachios and apricots.

STORAGE *Store covered containers in the refrigerator for up to 7 days.*

TIP *Rose water has an intoxicating, floral aroma, and just a little bit goes a long way. Major supermarkets usually carry it in the international foods aisle along with another favorite of mine, orange blossom water.*

Per Serving: Total calories: 275; Total fat: 12g; Saturated fat: 3g; Sodium: 72mg; Carbohydrates: 26g; Fiber: 3g; Protein: 19g

Breakfast Sweet Potatoes *with* Spiced Maple Yogurt *and* Walnuts

MAKES 4 SERVINGS

PREP TIME:
5 minutes

——

COOK TIME:
45 minutes

——

Sweet potatoes make surprisingly great breakfast items. They are packed with nutrients, including fiber, vitamin A, and vitamin C. Add Greek yogurt and walnuts, and you have a breakfast that will provide you with energy for hours.

4 red garnet sweet potatoes, about 6 inches long and 2 inches in diameter

2 cups low-fat (2%) plain Greek yogurt

¼ teaspoon pumpkin pie spice

1 tablespoon pure maple syrup

½ cup walnut pieces

1. Preheat the oven to 425°F. Line a sheet pan with a silicone baking mat or parchment paper.

2. Prick the sweet potatoes in multiple places with a fork and place on the sheet pan. Bake until tender when pricked with a paring knife, 40 to 45 minutes.

3. While the potatoes are baking, mix the yogurt, pumpkin pie spice, and maple syrup until well combined in a medium bowl.

4. When the potatoes are cool, slice the skin down the middle vertically to open up each potato. If you'd like to eat the sweet potatoes warm, place 1 potato in each of 4 containers and ½ cup of spiced yogurt plus 2 tablespoons of walnut pieces in each of 4 other containers. If you want to eat the potatoes cold, place ½ cup of yogurt and 2 tablespoons of walnuts directly on top of each of the 4 potatoes in the 4 containers.

STORAGE *Store covered containers in the refrigerator for up to 5 days.*

Per Serving: Total calories: 350; Total fat: 13g; Saturated fat: 3g; Sodium: 72mg; Carbohydrates: 46g; Fiber: 5g; Protein: 16g

Cocoa *and* Raspberry Overnight Oats

MAKES
5 SERVINGS

PREP TIME:
10 minutes

Chocolate and raspberries are a classic flavor combination and are delicious in oatmeal. The cocoa nibs are optional, but if your store carries them, add them for their roasted, somewhat bitter yet chocolaty crunch. If you need to make the oats gluten-free, just use certified gluten-free oats. Use cow's milk if you need to make this nut-free.

1²/₃ cups rolled oats

3¹/₃ cups unsweetened vanilla almond milk

2 teaspoons vanilla extract

1 tablespoon plus 2 teaspoons pure maple syrup

3 tablespoons chia seeds

3 tablespoons unsweetened cocoa powder

1²/₃ cups frozen raspberries

5 teaspoons cocoa nibs (optional)

1. In a large bowl, mix the oats, almond milk, vanilla, maple syrup, chia seeds, and cocoa powder until well combined.

2. Spoon ¾ cup of the oat mixture into each of 5 containers.

3. Top each serving with ⅓ cup of raspberries and 1 teaspoon of cocoa nibs, if using.

STORAGE *Store covered containers in the refrigerator for up to 5 days.*

TIP *Overnight oats can be eaten cold or reheated in the microwave.*

Per Serving: Total calories: 215; Total fat: 6g; Saturated fat: <1g; Sodium: 121mg; Carbohydrates: 34g; Fiber: 10g; Protein: 7g

Tahini Egg Salad *with* Pita

PREP TIME:
10 minutes

——

COOK TIME:
12 minutes

——

Egg salad is delicious mashed with tahini and fresh herbs. Tahini is highly nutritious and rich in B vitamins, antioxidants, and anti-inflammatory compounds. In place of the pita, you can also use lavash flatbread, crackers, or crispbread.

4 large eggs

¼ cup freshly chopped dill

**1 tablespoon plus
1 teaspoon unsalted tahini**

**2 teaspoons freshly
squeezed lemon juice**

⅛ teaspoon kosher salt

**4 whole-wheat
pitas, quartered**

1. Place the eggs in a saucepan and cover with water. Bring the water to a boil. As soon as the water starts to boil, place a lid on the pan and turn the heat off. Set a timer for 12 minutes.

2. When the timer goes off, drain the hot water and run cold water over the eggs to cool.

3. When the eggs are cool, peel them, place the yolks in a medium bowl, and mash them with a fork. Then chop the egg whites.

4. Add the chopped egg whites, dill, tahini, lemon juice (to taste), and salt to the bowl, and mix to combine.

5. Place a heaping ⅓ cup of egg salad in each of 4 containers. Place the pita in 4 separate containers or resealable bags so that the bread does not get soggy.

STORAGE *Store covered containers in the refrigerator for up to 5 days.*

TIP *Be sure to check the ingredient label of the tahini to make sure it is unsalted.*

Per Serving: Total calories: 242; Total fat: 10g; Saturated fat: 2g; Sodium: 300mg; Carbohydrates: 29g; Fiber: 5g; Protein: 13g

Super-Seed Granola

MAKES 8 SERVINGS

PREP TIME:
10 minutes

——

COOK TIME:
40 minutes

——

The serving size for most store-bought granola is only ¼ cup. The serving size for my super-seed granola is a hefty ½ cup, which, when paired with milk, a plant-based beverage, or yogurt, is hearty enough for breakfast and not just a crunchy garnish.

1½ cups rolled oats

⅓ cup raw quinoa

⅓ cup green pumpkin seeds (pepitas)

⅓ cup raw, unsalted sunflower seeds

2 tablespoons chia seeds

1 teaspoon ground cinnamon

⅓ cup pure maple syrup

⅓ cup unsweetened, unsalted sunflower seed butter

1. Preheat the oven to 325°F. Line a baking sheet with a silicone mat or parchment paper.

2. In a large mixing bowl, combine the oats, quinoa, pumpkin seeds, sunflower seeds, chia seeds, and cinnamon.

3. Place the maple syrup and sunflower seed butter in a small microwaveable bowl and microwave for 20 to 30 seconds to melt the seed butter. Pour it over the oat mixture and stir to coat.

4. Spread the granola evenly across the lined pan, bake for 15 minutes, stir, bake for 15 more minutes, stir, and bake for 10 more minutes. Remove the granola from the oven; it will get crunchier as it cools.

5. Place ½ cup of granola in each of 8 containers and store at room temperature.

STORAGE *Store covered containers at room temperature for 2 weeks.*

TIP *Sunflower seed butter is a fantastic alternative to nut or peanut butter. Green pumpkin seed butter is also an option you may be able to find in some stores.*

Per Serving: Total calories: 258; Total fat: 13g; Saturated fat: 1g; Sodium: 19mg; Carbohydrates: 30g; Fiber: 4g; Protein: 9g

Egg, Prosciutto, *and* Cheese Freezer Sandwiches

MAKES
6 SERVINGS

PREP TIME:
15 minutes

COOK TIME:
20 minutes

Breakfast sandwiches are fantastic meal prep, grab-and-go breakfast options, and they're even better when you can keep a stash in the freezer. Swiss cheese is a great ingredient, because it is significantly lower in sodium than other sliced cheeses.

Cooking spray or oil to grease the baking dish

7 large eggs

½ cup low-fat (2%) milk

½ teaspoon garlic powder

½ teaspoon onion powder

1 tablespoon Dijon mustard

½ teaspoon honey

6 whole-wheat English muffins

6 slices thinly sliced prosciutto

6 slices Swiss cheese

1. Preheat the oven to 375°F. Lightly oil or spray an 8-by-11-inch glass or ceramic baking dish with cooking spray.

2. In a large bowl, whisk together the eggs, milk, garlic powder, and onion powder. Pour the mixture into the baking dish and bake for 20 minutes, until the eggs are set and no longer jiggling. Cool.

3. While the eggs are baking, mix the mustard and honey in a small bowl. Lay out the English muffin halves to start assembly.

4. When the eggs are cool, use a biscuit cutter or drinking glass about the same size as the English muffin diameter to cut

6 egg circles. Divide the leftover egg scraps evenly to be added to each sandwich.

5. Spread ½ teaspoon of honey mustard on each of the bottom English muffin halves. Top each with 1 slice of prosciutto, 1 egg circle and scraps, 1 slice of cheese, and the top half of the muffin.

6. Wrap each sandwich tightly in foil.

STORAGE *Store tightly wrapped sandwiches in the freezer for up to 1 month. To reheat, remove the foil, place the sandwich on a microwave-safe plate, and wrap with a damp paper towel. Microwave on high for 1½ minutes, flip over, and heat again for another 1½ minutes. Because cooking time can vary greatly between microwaves, you may need to experiment with a few sandwiches before you find the perfect amount of time to heat the whole item through.*

TIP *If you have some extra veggies in the refrigerator, such as broccoli, cauliflower, or mushrooms, finely chop them and add them to the beaten eggs.*

Per Serving: Total calories: 361; Total fat: 17g; Saturated fat: 7g; Sodium: 953mg; Carbohydrates: 26g; Fiber: 3g; Protein: 24g

Farro Porridge *with* Blackberry Compote

PREP TIME:
5 minutes

———

COOK TIME:
30 minutes

———

Farro isn't a specific strain of wheat. It's actually a general term for wheat in Italian and can be spelt, emmer, or einkorn varieties, all of which are considered "ancient grains." You can use any of those products if you can't find farro.

FOR THE FARRO

1¼ cups uncooked semi-pearled farro

5 cups unsweetened vanilla almond milk

1 tablespoon pure maple syrup

FOR THE BLACKBERRY COMPOTE

1 (10-ounce) package frozen blackberries (2 cups)

2 teaspoons pure maple syrup

2 teaspoons balsamic vinegar

TO MAKE THE FARRO

1. Place the farro, almond milk, and maple syrup in a saucepan. Bring the liquid to a boil, then turn the heat down to low and simmer until the farro is tender and has absorbed much of the liquid, about 30 minutes. It should still look somewhat liquidy and will continue to absorb liquid as it cools.

2. Scoop ¾ cup of farro into each of 4 containers.

TO MAKE THE BLACKBERRY COMPOTE

3. While the farro is cooking, place the frozen blackberries, maple syrup, and balsamic vinegar in a separate saucepan on medium-low heat. Cook for 12 to 15 minutes, until the blackberry juices have thickened. Cool.

4. Spoon ¼ cup of the blackberry compote into each of the 4 farro containers.

STORAGE *Store covered containers in the refrigerator for up to 5 days.*

TIP *Purchasing farro can be a bit confusing, because the packages usually don't mention whether it is pearled or whole grain. Look at the recommended cooking time to tell the difference. Pearled usually takes about 10 minutes to cook, semi-pearled 20 to 30 minutes, and whole-grain about 40 minutes.*

Per Serving: Total calories: 334; Total fat: 5g; Saturated fat: 0g; Sodium: 227mg; Carbohydrates: 64g; Fiber: 11g; Protein: 11g

Egg, Feta, Spinach, *and* Artichoke Freezer Breakfast Burritos

MAKES 6 BURRITOS

PREP TIME:
15 minutes

COOK TIME:
5 minutes

The breakfast burrito is the perfect handheld, on-the-go vehicle for protein, veggies, and whole grains. I've taken healthy traditional Mediterranean flavors and put them into what is traditionally not a very healthy restaurant breakfast item.

8 large eggs

½ teaspoon dried Italian herbs

½ teaspoon garlic powder

½ teaspoon onion powder

3 teaspoons olive oil, divided

10 ounces baby spinach leaves

½ cup crumbled feta cheese

1 (14-ounce) can quartered artichoke hearts, super-tough leaves removed

6 (8- or 9-inch) whole-wheat tortillas

6 tablespoons prepared hummus or homemade hummus (see page 171)

1. Beat the eggs and whisk in the Italian herbs, garlic powder, and onion powder.

2. Heat 1 teaspoon of oil in a 12-inch skillet. When the oil is shimmering, add the spinach and sauté for 2 to 3 minutes, until the spinach is wilted. Remove the spinach from the pan.

3. In the same pan, heat the remaining 2 teaspoons of oil. When the oil is hot, add the eggs. When the eggs start to set, stir to scramble. Cook for about 3 minutes, then add the cooked spinach, feta, and artichoke hearts. Cool the mixture and pour off any liquid if it accumulates.

4. Place 1 tortilla on a cutting board. Spread 1 tablespoon of hummus down the middle of the tortilla. Place ¾ cup of the egg filling on top of the hummus. Fold the bottom end and sides over the filling and tightly roll up. Repeat for the remaining 5 tortillas.

5. Wrap each burrito in foil and place in a resealable plastic bag.

STORAGE *Store sealed bags in the freezer for up to 3 months. To reheat burritos, unwrap and remove the foil. Cover the burrito with a damp paper towel, place on a microwaveable plate, and microwave on high until the center of the burrito is hot, about 2 minutes.*

Per Serving: Total calories: 359; Total fat: 18g; Saturated fat: 6g; Sodium: 800mg; Carbohydrates: 32g; Fiber: 6g; Protein: 18g

Pumpkin, Apple, *and* Greek Yogurt Muffins

MAKES 12 MUFFINS

PREP TIME:
15 minutes

——

COOK TIME:
20 minutes

——

I love that 100 percent canned pumpkin is available all year long, not just during the fall! Greek yogurt is a great way to add extra protein, in addition to creating a moist muffin. Healthy fat comes in the form of olive oil, which you can use for baking.

Cooking spray to grease baking liners

2 cups whole-wheat flour

1 teaspoon aluminum-free baking powder (see tip on page 117)

1 teaspoon baking soda

⅛ teaspoon kosher salt

2 teaspoons ground cinnamon

½ teaspoon ground ginger

½ teaspoon ground allspice

⅔ cup pure maple syrup

1 cup low-fat (2%) plain Greek yogurt

1 cup 100% canned pumpkin

1 large egg

¼ cup extra-virgin olive oil

1½ cups chopped green apple (leave peel on)

½ cup walnut pieces

1. Preheat the oven to 400°F and line a muffin tin with 12 baking liners. Spray the liners lightly with cooking spray.

2. In a large bowl, whisk together the flour, baking powder, baking soda, salt, cinnamon, ginger, and allspice.

3. In a medium bowl, combine the maple syrup, yogurt, pumpkin, egg, olive oil, chopped apple, and walnuts.

4. Pour the wet ingredients into the dry ingredients and combine just until blended. Do not overmix.

5. Scoop about ¼ cup of batter into each muffin liner and bake for 20 minutes, or until the tops look browned and a paring knife comes out clean when inserted. Remove the muffins from the tin to cool.

TIP *If you've ever noticed a bitter taste in your baked goods, it could be because your baking powder contains aluminum. Be sure to use aluminum-free baking powder, which is available at some supermarkets, Trader Joe's, Whole Foods, and Sprouts.*

Per Serving: Total calories: 221; Total fat: 9g; Saturated fat: 1g; Sodium: 187mg; Carbohydrates: 32g; Fiber: 4g; Protein: 6g

Raspberry-Lemon Olive Oil Muffins

**MAKES
12 MUFFINS**

There is one cardinal rule in muffin making: Don't overmix the batter! For a moist muffin, be sure to mix the batter until just combined. If some streaks of flour remain, that's fine!

PREP TIME:
15 minutes

——

COOK TIME:
20 minutes

——

Cooking spray to grease baking liners

1 cup all-purpose flour

1 cup whole-wheat flour

½ cup tightly packed light brown sugar

½ teaspoon baking soda

½ teaspoon aluminum-free baking powder

⅛ teaspoon kosher salt

1¼ cups buttermilk

1 large egg

¼ cup extra-virgin olive oil

1 tablespoon freshly squeezed lemon juice

Zest of 2 lemons

1¼ cups frozen raspberries (do not thaw)

1. Preheat the oven to 400°F and line a muffin tin with 12 baking liners. Spray the liners lightly with cooking spray.

2. In a large mixing bowl, whisk together the all-purpose flour, whole-wheat flour, brown sugar, baking soda, baking powder, and salt.

3. In a medium bowl, whisk together the buttermilk, egg, oil, lemon juice, and lemon zest.

4. Pour the wet ingredients into the dry ingredients and stir just until blended. Do not overmix.

5. Fold in the frozen raspberries.

6. Scoop about ¼ cup of batter into each muffin liner and bake for 20 minutes, or until the tops look browned and a paring knife comes out clean when inserted. Remove the muffins from the tin to cool.

STORAGE *Store covered containers at room temperature for up to 4 days. To freeze muffins for up to 3 months, wrap them in foil and place in an airtight resealable bag.*

Per Serving: Total calories: 166; Total fat: 5g; Saturated fat: 1g; Sodium: 134mg; Carbohydrates: 30g; Fiber: 3g; Protein: 4g

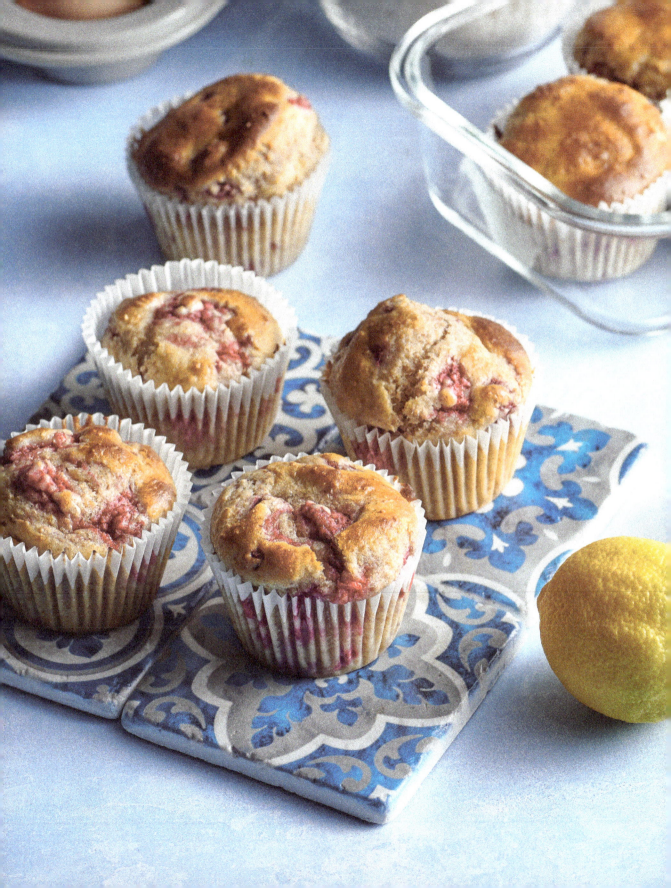

Savory Cucumber-Dill Yogurt

MAKES 4 SERVINGS

PREP TIME:
10 minutes
———

Change up your yogurt parfait game by making a savory version. The creamy, shallot-spiked yogurt goes very well with crunchy, cool cucumbers. This is a great way to add some veggies to your breakfast.

2 cups low-fat (2%) plain Greek yogurt

4 teaspoons minced shallot

4 teaspoons freshly squeezed lemon juice

¼ cup chopped fresh dill

2 teaspoons olive oil

¼ teaspoon kosher salt

Pinch freshly ground black pepper

2 cups chopped Persian cucumbers (about 4 medium cucumbers)

1. Combine the yogurt, shallot, lemon juice, dill, oil, salt, and pepper in a large bowl. Taste the mixture and add another pinch of salt if needed.

2. Scoop ½ cup of yogurt into each of 4 containers. Place ½ cup of chopped cucumbers in each of 4 separate small containers or resealable sandwich bags.

STORAGE *Store covered containers in the refrigerator for up to 5 days.*

TIP *The chopped cucumbers are stored separately because they will make the yogurt watery after a couple of days. Keeping them separate will also help them retain their crunch.*

Per Serving: Total calories: 127; Total fat: 5g; Saturated fat: 2g; Sodium: 200mg; Carbohydrates: 9g; Fiber: 2g; Protein: 11g

Strawberry-Mango Green Smoothie

**MAKES
2 SERVINGS**

PREP TIME:
10 minutes

———

Fruit is a major component of the Mediterranean diet, and making a smoothie is an easy way to consume it at breakfast or as a snack. If you have very sweet fruit, you may not need the honey, so taste the blended smoothie first, then add the honey if you need it. If you want the smoothie to be vegan, just use an unsweetened plant-based beverage, such as almond milk, soy milk, or coconut milk.

1½ cups low-fat (2%) milk

2 cups packed baby spinach leaves

½ cup sliced Persian or English cucumber, skin on

⅔ cup frozen strawberries

⅔ cup frozen mango chunks

1 medium very ripe banana, sliced (about ⅔ cup)

½ small avocado

1 teaspoon honey

1. Place the milk, spinach, cucumber, strawberries, mango, banana, and avocado in a blender.

2. Blend until smooth and taste. If the smoothie isn't sweet enough, add the honey.

3. Distribute the smoothie between 2 to-go cups.

STORAGE *Store smoothie cups in the refrigerator for up to 3 days.*

TIP *If using a traditional waxed cucumber, remove the peel.*

Per Serving: Total calories: 261; Total fat: 8g; Saturated fat: 2g; Sodium: 146mg; Carbohydrates: 40g; Fiber: 5g; Protein: 11g

Pepper, Kale, *and* Chickpea Shakshuka

PREP TIME:
15 minutes

———

COOK TIME:
35 minutes

———

This is not your traditional shakshuka. My version is less saucy and more textural, with veggies and chickpeas to keep you fuller longer. You'll definitely make a dent in your daily quota of veggies at breakfast.

1 tablespoon olive oil

1 small red onion, thinly sliced

1 red bell pepper, thinly sliced

1 green bell pepper, thinly sliced

1 bunch kale, stemmed and roughly chopped

½ cup packed cilantro leaves, chopped

½ teaspoon kosher salt

1 teaspoon smoked paprika

1 (14.5-ounce) can diced tomatoes

1 (14-ounce) can low-sodium chickpeas, drained and rinsed

⅔ cup water

5 eggs

2½ whole-wheat pitas (optional)

1. Preheat the oven to 375°F.
2. Heat the oil in an oven-safe 12-inch skillet over medium-high heat. Once the oil is shimmering, add the onions and red and green bell peppers. Sauté for 5 minutes, then cover, leaving the lid slightly ajar. Cook for 5 more minutes, then add the kale and cover, leaving the lid slightly ajar. Cook for 10 more minutes, stirring occasionally.
3. Add the cilantro, salt, paprika, tomatoes, chickpeas, and water, and stir to combine.
4. Make 5 wells in the mixture. Break an egg into a small bowl and pour it into a well. Repeat with the remaining 4 eggs.

5. Place the pan in the oven and bake until the egg whites are opaque and the eggs still jiggle a little when the pan is shaken, about 12 to 15 minutes, but start checking at 8 minutes.

6. When the shakshuka is cool, scoop about 1¼ cups of veggies into each of 5 containers, along with 1 egg each. If using, place ½ pita in each of 5 resealable bags.

STORAGE *Store covered containers in the refrigerator for up to 5 days.*

TIP *Remember that the eggs will continue to cook when reheated. Keep that in mind when deciding when to remove the shakshuka from the oven.*

Per Serving: Total calories: 244; Total fat: 9g; Saturated fat: 2g; Sodium: 529mg; Carbohydrates: 29g; Fiber: 8g; Protein: 14g

Whole-Wheat Pancakes *with* Spiced Peach *and* Orange Compote

**MAKES
6 SERVINGS**

PREP TIME:
15 minutes

———

COOK TIME:
15 minutes

———

Pancakes are great meal prep breakfast items, because they reheat exceptionally well and keep their integrity. Greek yogurt makes these pancakes extra moist. I've replaced traditional maple syrup with a fruit-juice-sweetened peach compote with just a hint of spice.

FOR THE PANCAKES

1½ cups whole-wheat flour

1 teaspoon baking powder

½ teaspoon baking soda

½ teaspoon ground cinnamon

⅛ teaspoon kosher salt

1 large egg

1 cup low-fat (2%) plain Greek yogurt

1 tablespoon honey

1 cup low-fat (2%) milk

2 teaspoons olive oil, divided

FOR THE COMPOTE

1 (10-ounce) package frozen sliced peaches

½ cup orange juice

¼ teaspoon pumpkin pie spice

TO MAKE THE PANCAKES

1. Combine the flour, baking powder, baking soda, cinnamon, and salt in a large mixing bowl and whisk to make sure everything is distributed evenly. In a separate bowl, whisk together the egg, yogurt, honey, and milk. Pour the liquid ingredients into the dry ingredients and stir until just combined. Do not overmix.

2. Heat ½ teaspoon of oil in a 12-inch skillet or griddle over medium heat. Once the pan is hot, spoon ¼ cup of pancake batter into the pan. You should be able to fit 3 pancakes

in a 12-inch skillet. Cook each side for about 1 minute and 30 seconds, watching carefully and checking the underside for a golden but not burnt color before flipping. Repeat until all the batter has been used.

3. Place 2 pancakes in each of 6 containers.

TO MAKE THE COMPOTE

4. Thaw the peaches in the microwave just to the point that they can be cut, about 30 seconds on high. Cut the peaches into 1-inch pieces.

5. Bring the peaches, orange juice, and pumpkin pie spice to a boil in a saucepan. As soon as bubbles appear, lower the heat to medium-low and cook for 12 minutes, until the juice has thickened and the peaches are very soft. Allow to cool, then mash with a potato masher.

6. Place 2 tablespoons of compote in each of 6 sauce containers.

STORAGE *Store covered pancake containers in the refrigerator for up to 5 days or in the freezer for up to 2 months. Peach compote will last up to 2 weeks in the refrigerator and up to 2 months in the freezer.*

Per Serving: Total calories: 209; Total fat: 5g; Saturated fat: 2g; Sodium: 289mg; Carbohydrates: 34g; Fiber: 4g; Protein: 11g

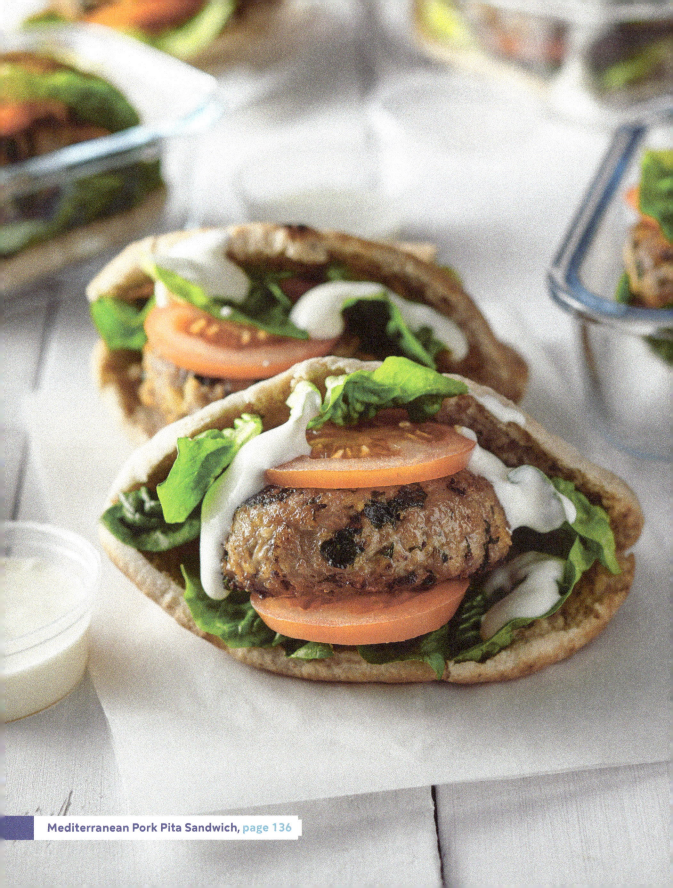

CHAPTER 10

Lunch *and* Dinner

Balsamic Chicken *and* Veggie Skewers

PREP TIME:
20 minutes,
plus 2 hours
to marinate

———

COOK TIME:
25 minutes

———

You don't need a grill to make chicken and veggie skewers. Baking in a 450°F oven ensures that everything gets cooked through, but the veggies stay crisp-tender. Removing the stems from the mushrooms makes it easier to slide them onto the skewers without breaking them.

1 pound boneless, skinless chicken breasts, cut into 1-inch cubes

⅓ cup balsamic vinegar

4 tablespoons olive oil, divided

4 teaspoons dried Italian herbs, divided

2 teaspoons garlic powder, divided

2 teaspoons onion powder, divided

8 ounces whole button or cremini mushrooms, stems removed

1 large red bell pepper, cut into 1-inch squares

1 small red onion, quartered and layers pulled apart

1 large zucchini, sliced into ½-inch rounds

¾ teaspoon kosher salt

8 (11¾-inch) wooden or metal skewers, soaked in water for at least 1 hour if wooden

1. Preheat the oven to 450°F. Line a sheet pan with aluminum foil.

2. Place the chicken in a gallon-size resealable bag along with the balsamic vinegar, 2 tablespoons of oil, 2 teaspoons of Italian herbs, 1 teaspoon of garlic powder, and 1 teaspoon of onion powder. Seal the bag and make sure all the pieces of chicken are coated with marinade.

3. In a second resealable bag, place the mushrooms, bell pepper, onion, and zucchini and the remaining 2 tablespoons of oil, 2 teaspoons of Italian herbs, 1 teaspoon of garlic powder, and 1 teaspoon of onion powder. Seal the bag and shake to make sure the veggies are coated.

4. Refrigerate both bags and marinate for at least 2 hours.

5. Thread the chicken and veggies on 8 skewers, alternating both chicken and veggies on each skewer. Place 6 skewers vertically in the center of the pan, 1 horizontally at the top, and 1 at the bottom. Sprinkle half the salt over the skewers, then flip over and sprinkle the skewers with the remaining salt.

6. Bake for 15 minutes, carefully flip the skewers, then bake for another 10 minutes. Cool.

7. If you have containers long enough to fit the skewers, place 2 skewers directly in each of 4 containers. If not, break the skewers in half or slide the meat and veggies off the skewers.

STORAGE *Store covered containers in the refrigerator for up to 5 days.*

TIP *Soaking wooden skewers is essential when baking or grilling with them. This step will ensure they do not catch on fire during the cooking process.*

Per Serving: Total calories: 224; Total fat: 10g; Saturated fat: 2g; Sodium: 631mg; Carbohydrates: 11g; Fiber: 3g; Protein: 27g

Baked Chicken Thighs *with* Lemon, Olives, *and* Brussels Sprouts

MAKES 4 SERVINGS

PREP TIME:
10 minutes
—

COOK TIME:
40 minutes
—

Dark meat gets a bad rap nutritionally speaking. While it has a little bit more fat and calories, it actually contains more iron and zinc than white meat. Thigh meat doesn't overcook as easily as chicken breasts, which allows a longer baking time to ensure that the veggies are cooked through. Serve this dish with Bulgur Pilaf with Almonds (page 196).

2 tablespoons olive oil, divided

1 pound Brussels sprouts, stemmed and halved (quartered if the sprouts are extra large)

1 pound boneless, skinless chicken thighs

2 teaspoons chopped garlic

1 teaspoon dried oregano

½ teaspoon kosher salt

3 tablespoons freshly squeezed lemon juice

½ cup pitted kalamata olives

1. Preheat the oven to 350°F.

2. Spread 1 tablespoon of oil over the bottom of a 13-by-9-inch glass or ceramic baking dish. Add the Brussels sprouts to the pan and spread out evenly. Place the chicken on top of the sprouts and rub the garlic and oregano into the top of the chicken.

3. Sprinkle the salt, the remaining 1 tablespoon of oil, the lemon juice, and the olives over the contents of the pan.

4. Cover the pan with aluminum foil and bake for 20 minutes. Remove the foil and bake uncovered for 20 more minutes. Cool.

5. Place one quarter of the chicken and ¾ cup of Brussels sprouts in each of 4 containers. Drizzle any remaining juices from the pan over the chicken.

STORAGE *Store covered containers in the refrigerator for 5 days.*

Per Serving: Total calories: 287; Total fat: 18g; Saturated fat: 3g; Sodium: 737mg; Carbohydrates: 14g; Fiber: 5g; Protein: 20g

Mediterranean-Style Pesto Chicken

MAKES
4 SERVINGS

PREP TIME:
15 minutes,
plus
1 hour for
marinating
——

COOK TIME:
40 minutes
——

Prepared pesto is such a flavorful and handy convenience item. The saltiness of the pesto works well with the acidity of the Chunky Roasted Cherry Tomato and Basil Sauce (page 174), which is actually thick enough to work as a compote. If you need a starch to round out your meal, add something simple, such as Garlic-Chive Quinoa (see page 44).

1 pound chicken breasts (2 large breasts), butterflied and cut in half to make 4 pieces

1 (6-ounce) jar prepared pesto

1 teaspoon olive oil

12 ounces baby spinach leaves

Chunky Roasted Cherry Tomato and Basil Sauce (page 174)

1. Place the chicken and pesto in a gallon-size resealable bag. Marinate for at least 1 hour.

2. Preheat the oven to 350°F and rub a 13-by-9-inch glass or ceramic baking dish with the oil, or spray with cooking spray.

3. Place the spinach in the pan, then place the chicken on top of the spinach. Pour the pesto from the bag into the dish. Cover the pan with aluminum foil and bake for 20 minutes. Remove the foil and bake for another 15 to 20 minutes. Cool.

4. Place 1 piece of chicken, one quarter of the spinach, and ⅓ cup of chunky tomato sauce in each of 4 separate containers.

STORAGE *Store covered containers in the refrigerator for up to 5 days.*

TIP *If you don't want to butterfly large chicken breasts to turn them into more manageable portion sizes that cook evenly, buy chicken labeled "thin-sliced breast fillets."*

Per Serving: Total calories: 531; Total fat: 43g; Saturated fat: 7g; Sodium: 1,243mg; Carbohydrates: 13g; Fiber: 4g; Protein: 29g

Italian-Inspired Rotisserie Chicken _and_ Broccoli Slaw

**MAKES
4 SERVINGS**

PREP TIME:
15 minutes

Salads without lettuce can be a great way to mix up your salad routine. Broccoli slaw provides tons of crunch and adds a very important phytonutrient called sulforaphane that may help prevent cancer. If your supermarket doesn't carry broccoli slaw, you can also use a cabbage-based slaw.

4 cups packaged broccoli slaw

1 cooked rotisserie chicken, meat removed (about 10 to 12 ounces)

1 bunch red radishes, stemmed, halved, and thickly sliced (about 1¼ cups)

1 cup sliced red onion

½ cup pitted kalamata or niçoise olives, roughly chopped

½ cup sliced pepperoncini

8 tablespoons Dijon Red Wine Vinaigrette (page 177), divided

1. Place the broccoli slaw, chicken, radishes, onion, olives, and pepperoncini in a large mixing bowl. Toss to combine.
2. Place 2½ cups of salad in each of 4 containers. Pour 2 tablespoons of vinaigrette into each of 4 sauce containers.

STORAGE _Store covered containers in the refrigerator for up to 5 days._

TIP _If you do your vegetable prep the day before actually cooking the meals, store your sliced radishes in a container of cold water so that they stay crisp and retain their color._

Per Serving: Total calories: 329; Total fat: 24g; Saturated fat: 4g; Sodium: 849mg; Carbohydrates: 10g; Fiber: 3g; Protein: 20g

Herbed Tuna Salad Wraps

MAKES 4 SERVINGS

PREP TIME:
15 minutes

———

These tuna salad wraps are great when you're in the mood for a light and refreshing lunch with lots of crunch. Packed with nutrients, such as iron, zinc, and vitamins A, C, B$_6$, and D, this recipe puts you well on your way to meeting your daily micronutrient needs.

1 (11-ounce) pouch tuna in water

1 cup parsley leaves, chopped

¼ cup mint leaves, chopped

¼ cup minced shallot

1½ teaspoons sumac

1 teaspoon Dijon mustard

1 tablespoon olive oil

1 tablespoon freshly squeezed lemon juice

¼ cup unsalted sunflower seeds

16 large or medium romaine or bibb lettuce leaves

1 red bell pepper, cut into thin sticks (3 to 4 inches long)

3 Persian cucumbers, cut into thin sticks (3 to 4 inches long)

1. In a large bowl, mix together the tuna, parsley, mint, shallot, sumac, mustard, oil, lemon juice, and sunflower seeds.
2. Place ¾ cup of tuna salad in each of 4 containers. Place 4 lettuce leaves, one quarter of the peppers, and one quarter of the cucumbers in each of 4 separate containers so that they don't get soggy from the tuna salad.

STORAGE *Store covered containers in the refrigerator for up to 4 days.*

TIP *Tuna in pouches is preferable to cans, because pouches don't need to be drained and the tuna isn't soggy. You can substitute canned salmon, canned sardines, or even shredded rotisserie chicken for the tuna in this salad.*

Per Serving: Total calories: 223; Total fat: 9g; Saturated fat: 1g; Sodium: 422mg; Carbohydrates: 12g; Fiber: 4g; Protein: 24g

Chicken Sausage, Artichoke, Kale, *and* White Bean Gratin

**MAKES
8 SERVINGS**

*Chicken sausage, beans, and veggies make up this hearty
casserole. The soft goat cheese adds a tangy creaminess,
while the wine adds a touch of acidity.*

PREP TIME:
15 minutes

——

COOK TIME:
45 minutes

——

**2 teaspoons olive oil, plus
2 tablespoons**

**1 small yellow onion,
chopped (about 2 cups)**

**1 (12-ounce) package fully
cooked chicken-apple
sausage, sliced**

**1 bunch kale, stemmed and
chopped (6 to 7 cups)**

**½ cup dry white wine, such
as sauvignon blanc**

4 ounces soft goat cheese

**2 (15.5-ounce) cans
cannellini or great northern
beans, drained and rinsed**

**1 (14-ounce) can quartered
artichoke hearts**

**1 (14.5-ounce) can no-salt-
added diced tomatoes**

**1 teaspoon herbes
de Provence**

¼ teaspoon kosher salt

1 cup panko bread crumbs

1 teaspoon garlic powder

1. Preheat the oven to 350°F. Lightly oil a 13-by-9-inch glass or
   ceramic baking dish.

2. Heat 2 teaspoons of oil in a 12-inch skillet over medium-high
   heat. When the oil is shimmering, add the onion and cook for
   2 minutes. Add the sausage and brown for 3 minutes. Add the
   kale and cook until wilted, about 3 more minutes. Add the wine
   and cook for 1 additional minute.

3. Add the goat cheese and stir until it is melted and the
   mixture looks creamy.

4. Add the beans, artichokes, tomatoes, herbes de Provence,
   and salt, and stir to combine. Transfer the contents of the pan
   to the baking dish.

5. Mix the bread crumbs, the garlic powder, and the remaining
   2 tablespoons of oil in a small bowl. Spread the bread crumbs
   evenly across the top of the casserole.

6. Cover the dish with foil and bake for 30 minutes. Remove the foil and bake for 15 more minutes, until the bread crumbs are lightly browned. Cool.

7. Place about 1½ cups of casserole in each of 8 containers.

STORAGE *Store covered containers in the refrigerator for up to 5 days. Gratin can be frozen for up to 3 months.*

TIP *You can use other flavors of chicken sausage, including Italian, spicy, or spinach-and-feta varieties.*

Per Serving: Total calories: 367; Total fat: 14g; Saturated fat: 5g; Sodium: 624mg; Carbohydrates: 40g; Fiber: 10g; Protein: 19g

Mediterranean Pork Pita Sandwich

MAKES 6 SANDWICHES

PREP TIME:
15 minutes

———

COOK TIME:
10 minutes

———

The flavorful and tender pork patty for this pita sandwich is very versatile, because you can also use it as a burger or on top of a salad, or you can even roll the filling into meatballs. You can also use different veggies as toppings, such as spinach leaves, sliced cucumbers, sliced peppers, radishes, and red onion.

2 teaspoons olive oil, plus 1 tablespoon

2 cups packed baby spinach leaves, finely chopped

4 ounces mushrooms, finely chopped

1 teaspoon chopped garlic

1 pound extra-lean ground pork

1 large egg

½ cup panko bread crumbs

⅓ cup chopped fresh dill

¼ teaspoon kosher salt

6 large romaine lettuce leaves, ripped into pieces to fit pita

2 tomatoes, sliced

3 whole-wheat pitas, cut in half

¾ cup Garlic Yogurt Sauce (page 165)

1. Heat 2 teaspoons of oil in a 12-inch skillet over medium heat. Once the oil is shimmering, add the spinach, mushrooms, and garlic and sauté for 3 minutes. Cool for 5 minutes.

2. Place the mushroom mixture in a large mixing bowl and add the pork, egg, bread crumbs, dill, and salt. Mix with your hands until everything is well combined. Make 6 patties, about ½-inch thick and 3 inches in diameter.

3. Heat the remaining 1 tablespoon of oil in the same 12-inch skillet over medium-high heat. When the oil is hot, add the patties. They should all be able to fit in the pan. If not, cook in 2 batches. Cook for 5 minutes on the first side and 4 minutes on the second side. The outside should be golden brown, and the inside should no longer be pink.

4. Place 1 patty in each of 6 containers. In each of 6 separate containers that will not be reheated, place 1 torn lettuce leaf and 2 tomato slices. Wrap the pita halves in plastic wrap and place one in each veggie container. Spoon 2 tablespoons of yogurt sauce into each of 6 sauce containers.

STORAGE *Store covered containers in the refrigerator for up to 5 days. Uncooked patties can be frozen for up to 4 months, while cooked patties can be frozen for up to 3 months.*

TIP *Use extra-lean pork, not the 80% lean/20% fat type. There's too much grease when cooking the patties. If you can't find extra-lean ground pork, use ground turkey or chicken.*

Per Serving: Total calories: 309; Total fat: 11g; Saturated fat: 3g; Sodium: 343mg; Carbohydrates: 22g; Fiber: 3g; Protein: 32g

Greek-Style Braised Pork *with* Leeks, Greens, *and* Potatoes

**MAKES
4 SERVINGS**

This hearty dish is designed to resemble a Mediterranean version of a pork chili verde. It's a one-pot meal that provides protein, veggies, and starch. Adding potatoes means you don't need to make a separate starch side, such as rice.

PREP TIME:
20 minutes

———

COOK TIME:
1 hour
40 minutes

———

1 tablespoon olive oil, plus 2 teaspoons

1¼ pounds boneless pork loin chops, fat cap removed and cut into 1-inch pieces

2 leeks, white and light green parts quartered vertically and thinly sliced

1 bulb fennel, quartered and thinly sliced

1 cup chopped onion

1 teaspoon chopped garlic

2 cups reduced-sodium chicken broth

1 teaspoon fennel seed

1 teaspoon dried oregano

½ teaspoon kosher salt

1 pound baby red potatoes, halved

1 bunch chard, including stems, chopped

2 tablespoons freshly squeezed lemon juice

1. Heat 1 tablespoon of oil in a soup pot or Dutch oven over medium-high heat. When the oil is shimmering, add the pork cubes and brown for about 6 minutes, turning the cubes over after 3 minutes. Remove the pork to a plate.

2. Add the remaining 2 teaspoons of oil to the same pot and add the leeks, fennel, onion, and garlic. Cook for 3 minutes.

3. Pour the broth into the pan, scraping up any browned bits on the bottom. Add the fennel seed, oregano, and salt, and add the pork, plus any juices that may have accumulated on the plate. Make sure the pork is submerged in the liquid. Place the potatoes on top, then place the chard on top of the potatoes.

4. Cover, turn down the heat to low, and simmer for 1½ hours, until the pork is tender. When the pork is done cooking, add the lemon juice. Taste and add more salt if needed. Cool.

5. Scoop 2 cups of the mixture into each of 4 containers.

Store covered containers in the refrigerator for up to 5 days.

TIP *Boneless loin chops work well because they're already cut to an even thickness, but you can also use pork loin or tenderloin. The amount called for is just a little over a pound to account for the visible fat that you will probably need to remove.*

Per Serving: Total calories: 378; Total fat: 13g; Saturated fat: 3g; Sodium: 1,607mg; Carbohydrates: 33g; Fiber: 8g; Protein: 34g

Slow Cooker Lamb, Herb, *and* Bean Stew

MAKES 4 SERVINGS

PREP TIME:
20 minutes

———

COOK TIME:
15 minutes
on the
stovetop,
plus 8 hours
in the
slow cooker

———

This stew is jam-packed with herbs! Parsley is more than just a garnish here. It makes up the base of this comforting stew. Parsley has an impressive nutrient profile, including a range of disease-fighting antioxidants, such as lutein, which is essential for good eye health. Cooking this stew in the slow cooker produces super-tender meat without having to heat up the kitchen for hours. Serve with Garlic-Chive Quinoa (see page 44) or Roasted Spaghetti Squash (see page 29).

3 bunches of parsley (about 6 packed cups of leaves)

1 large bunch cilantro (about 1½ packed cups of leaves)

1 bunch scallions, sliced (both white and green parts, about 1¼ cups)

1 pound leg of lamb, fat trimmed, cut into 1-inch pieces

2 tablespoons olive oil, divided

1 medium onion, chopped

2 teaspoons chopped garlic

2 teaspoons turmeric

¾ teaspoon kosher salt

2 tablespoons tomato paste

2½ cups low-sodium chicken broth

2 (15.5-ounce) cans low-sodium kidney beans, drained and rinsed

2 tablespoons freshly squeezed lemon juice

1. Finely chop the parsley leaves, cilantro leaves, and scallions with a knife, or pulse in the food processor until finely chopped but not puréed. With this amount of herbs, you'll need to pulse in two batches.

2. Pat the lamb cubes with a paper towel. Heat a 12-inch skillet over medium-high heat and add 1 tablespoon of oil. Once the oil is shimmering, add the lamb and brown for 5 minutes, flipping after 3 minutes. Place the lamb in the slow cooker.

3. Turn the heat down to medium and add the remaining 1 tablespoon of oil to the skillet. Once the oil is hot, add the onions and garlic and sauté for 3 minutes. Add the turmeric, salt, and tomato paste and continue to cook for 2 more minutes, stirring frequently.

4. Add the chopped parsley, cilantro, and scallions. Sauté for 5 minutes, stirring occasionally.

5. While the herbs are cooking, add the broth, beans, and lemon juice to the slow cooker. Add the herb mixture when it's done cooking on the stove. Turn the slow cooker to the low setting and cook for 8 hours.

6. Taste and add more salt and/or lemon juice if needed. Cool.

7. Scoop 2 cups of stew into each of 4 containers.

STORAGE *Store covered containers in the refrigerator for up to 5 days. Stew can be frozen for up to 4 months.*

TIP *If you're not a lamb fan, beef works very well with this recipe.*

Per Serving: Total calories: 486; Total fat: 15g; Saturated fat: 5g; Sodium: 690mg; Carbohydrates: 51g; Fiber: 15g; Protein: 41g

Beef *and* Veggie Lasagna

**MAKES
10 SERVINGS**

PREP TIME:
15 minutes

——

COOK TIME:
1 hour
10 minutes

——

I can't think of many meals more comforting than a big piece of lasagna. Beef is more of an accessory in this version in order to make room for more veggies. If you don't want to chop the mushrooms by hand, you can pulse them in a food processor.

3 teaspoons olive oil, divided

1 medium zucchini, quartered lengthwise and chopped (about 1⅓ cups)

3 cups packed baby spinach

1 cup chopped yellow onion

1 teaspoon chopped garlic

8 ounces button or cremini mushrooms, finely chopped

1 cup shredded carrots

8 ounces lean (90/10) ground beef

½ cup dry red wine

1 (28-ounce) can low-sodium or no-salt-added crushed tomatoes

1 (15-ounce) can tomato sauce

¼ teaspoon kosher salt

1 (16-ounce) container low-fat (2%) cottage cheese

1 large egg

3 tablespoons grated Parmesan cheese

2 cups shredded part-skim mozzarella cheese, divided

½ cup fresh basil leaves, chopped

1 (9-ounce) box oven-ready lasagna noodles

1. Preheat the oven to 375°F.
2. Heat 1 teaspoon of oil in a 12-inch skillet over medium-high heat. When the oil is shimmering, add the zucchini and cook for 2 minutes. Add the spinach and continue to cook for 1 more minute. Remove the veggies to a plate.
3. In the same skillet, heat the remaining 2 teaspoons of oil over medium-high heat. When the oil is hot, add the onion and garlic and cook for 2 minutes. Add the mushrooms and

carrots and cook for 4 more minutes. Add the ground beef and continue cooking for 4 more minutes, until the meat has browned. Add the wine and cook for 1 minute. Add the crushed tomatoes, tomato sauce, and salt, stir, and turn off the heat.

4. In a large mixing bowl, combine the cottage cheese, egg, and Parmesan, ½ cup of shredded cheese, and the basil.

5. Ladle 2 cups of sauce on the bottom of a 9-by-13-inch glass or ceramic baking dish. Place 4 noodles side by side in the pan. Layer 1 cup of sauce, half of the veggies, and half of the cottage cheese. Repeat with 4 more noodles, 1 cup of sauce, the remaining half of the veggies, and the remaining half of the cottage cheese. Top with 4 more noodles, the remainder of the sauce, and the remaining 1½ cups of shredded cheese.

6. Cover the pan with foil, trying not to touch the foil to the cheese, and bake for 40 minutes. Remove the foil and bake for 10 to 15 more minutes, until the cheese starts to brown.

7. When the lasagna cools, cut it into 10 pieces and place 1 piece in each of 10 containers.

STORAGE *Store covered containers in the refrigerator for up to 5 days. Cooked lasagna freezes well and can last for up to 3 months.*

TIP *If you tightly cover the pan with foil, the cheese will stick to the foil. Tent two pieces of foil horizontally across the pan so that the cheese won't stick.*

Per Serving: Total calories: 321; Total fat: 11g; Saturated fat: 4g; Sodium: 680mg; Carbohydrates: 34g; Fiber: 5g; Protein: 24g

Moroccan Spiced Stir-Fried Beef *with* Butternut Squash *and* Chickpeas

MAKES 4 SERVINGS

PREP TIME:
15 minutes

COOK TIME:
15 minutes

Beef tagine is a traditional Moroccan dish, but it can take a long time to cook. This quickly cooked beef uses the same flavors as a tagine, in addition to butternut squash, chickpeas, cilantro, dried apricots, and almonds. Don't skip the baking-soda soak step, because it makes the beef strips extra tender.

1 tablespoon olive oil, plus 2 teaspoons

1 pound precut butternut squash cut into ½-inch cubes

3 ounces scallions, white and green parts chopped (1 cup)

1 tablespoon water

¼ teaspoon baking soda

¾ pound flank steak, sliced across the grain into ⅛-inch thick slices

½ teaspoon garlic powder

¼ teaspoon ground ginger

¼ teaspoon turmeric

¼ teaspoon ground cumin

¼ teaspoon ground coriander

⅛ teaspoon cayenne pepper

⅛ teaspoon ground cinnamon

½ teaspoon kosher salt, divided

1 (14-ounce) can chickpeas, drained and rinsed

½ cup dried apricots, quartered

½ cup cilantro leaves, chopped

2 teaspoons freshly squeezed lemon juice

8 teaspoons sliced almonds

1. Heat 1 tablespoon of oil in a 12-inch skillet. Once the oil is hot, add the squash and scallions, and cook until the squash is tender, about 10 to 12 minutes.

2. Mix the water and baking soda together in a small prep bowl. Place the beef in a medium bowl, pour the baking-soda water over it, and mix to combine. Let it sit for 5 minutes.

3. In a small bowl, combine the garlic powder, ginger, turmeric, cumin, coriander, cayenne, cinnamon, and ¼ teaspoon of salt, then add the mixture to the beef. Stir to combine.

4. When the squash is tender, turn the heat off and add the remaining ¼ teaspoon of salt and the chickpeas, dried apricots, cilantro, and lemon juice to taste. Stir to combine. Place the contents of the pan in a bowl to cool.

5. Clean out the skillet and heat the remaining 2 teaspoons of oil over high heat. When the oil is hot, add the beef and cook until it is no longer pink, about 2 to 3 minutes.

6. Place 1¼ cups of the squash mixture and one quarter of the beef slices in each of 4 containers. Sprinkle 2 teaspoons of sliced almonds over each container.

STORAGE *Store covered containers in the refrigerator for up to 5 days.*

TIP *Some precut squash is sold in 1-inch pieces. Be sure to cut those in half so that the cooking time stays below 15 minutes.*

Per Serving: Total calories: 404; Total fat: 14g; Saturated fat: 1g; Sodium: 355mg; Carbohydrates: 46g; Fiber: 12g; Protein: 27g

Red Wine–Braised Pot Roast
with Carrots *and* Mushrooms

**MAKES
4 SERVINGS**

PREP TIME:
15 minutes

———

COOK TIME:
25 minutes
on the
stovetop,
plus
3 hours in
the oven

———

Pot roast cooked with red wine is a treat during the winter on a chilly day. The vegetables not only give flavor to the sauce but also serve as your veggie side. Serve with Creamy Polenta with Chives and Parmesan (page 195) for the ultimate comfort-food dish. Freeze the extra meat if you can't find a roast close to 1 pound.

1 pound tri-tip roast

¼ teaspoon kosher salt

1 tablespoon olive oil

2 cups chopped onion

1 teaspoon chopped garlic

3 medium carrots, cut into ½-inch pieces (2 cups)

2 large celery stalks, cut into ½-inch pieces (1 cup)

8 ounces button or cremini mushrooms, halved

½ teaspoon fennel seed

½ teaspoon dried thyme

½ teaspoon dried oregano

1 (14.5-ounce) can no-salt-added diced tomatoes

1 cup dry red wine, such as red zinfandel or cabernet sauvignon

1 cup reduced-sodium beef broth

1. Preheat the oven to 325°F.

2. Season the roast with the salt.

3. Heat the oil in a Dutch oven or heavy-bottomed soup pot over high heat. Once the oil is hot, add the roast and brown for 3 minutes on each side. Remove the roast to a plate.

4. Add the onion, garlic, carrots, celery, and mushrooms to the pot and cook for 5 minutes.

5. Add the fennel seed, thyme, oregano, tomatoes, red wine, and broth and bring to a simmer. Cover the pot with a tight-fitting lid or foil and place in the oven. Cook until the meat is very tender, about 3 hours.

6. Remove the roast to a plate and spoon the vegetables into a bowl with a slotted spoon. Place the pot on high heat and reduce the liquid by half, about 10 minutes. If your pot is extra wide, it will take less time for the liquid to reduce. Add more salt if needed.

7. After the meat has cooled, cut 12 slices against the grain. Place 3 slices, ¾ cup of vegetables, and ⅓ cup of sauce in each of 4 containers.

STORAGE *Store covered containers in the refrigerator for up to 5 days.*

TIP *If you can't find a tri-tip roast at the supermarket, alternative beef cuts that can be used are brisket, boneless chuck roast, or bottom round. When in doubt, tell the butcher you're making pot roast, and they will know what you need.*

Per Serving: Total calories: 366; Total fat: 14g; Saturated fat: 4g; Sodium: 468mg; Carbohydrates: 23g; Fiber: 6g; Protein: 28g

North African–Inspired Sautéed Shrimp *with* Leeks *and* Peppers

**MAKES
4 SERVINGS**

PREP TIME:
15 minutes

———

COOK TIME:
20 minutes

———

I took the flavors of a chermoula sauce—which is popular in Morocco, Algeria, and Tunisia—and used them as the seasoning for this dish. Taste before adding salt, because you may find that you don't need it. You can serve this dish with Orange and Cinnamon–Scented Whole-Wheat Couscous (page 194) or with more hearty grains like farro and kamut.

2 tablespoons olive oil, divided

1 large leek, white and light green parts, halved lengthwise, sliced ¼-inch thick

2 teaspoons chopped garlic

1 large red bell pepper, chopped into ¼-inch pieces

1 cup chopped fresh parsley leaves (1 small bunch)

½ cup chopped fresh cilantro leaves (½ small bunch)

¼ teaspoon ground cumin

¼ teaspoon ground coriander

1 teaspoon smoked paprika

1 pound uncooked peeled, deveined large shrimp (20 to 25 per pound), thawed if frozen, blotted with paper towels

1 tablespoon freshly squeezed lemon juice

⅛ teaspoon kosher salt

1. Heat 2 teaspoons of oil in a 12-inch skillet over medium heat. Once the oil is hot, add the leeks and garlic and sauté for 2 minutes. Add the peppers and cook for 10 minutes, or until the peppers are soft, stirring occasionally.

2. Add the chopped parsley and cilantro and cook for 1 more minute. Remove the mixture from the pan and place in a medium bowl.

3. Mix the cumin, coriander, and paprika in a small prep bowl.

Continued »

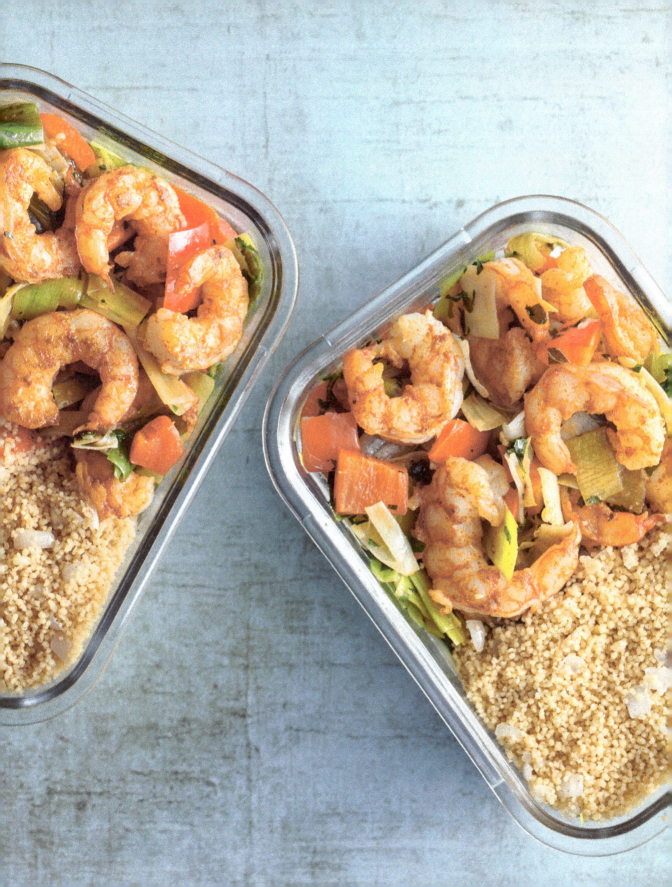

4. Add 2 teaspoons of oil to the same skillet and increase the heat to medium-high. Add the shrimp in a single layer, sprinkle the spice mixture over the shrimp, and cook for about 2 minutes. Flip the shrimp over and cook for 1 more minute. Add the leek and herb mixture, stir, and cook for 1 more minute.

5. Turn off the heat and add the remaining 2 teaspoons of oil and the lemon juice. Taste to see whether you need the salt. Add if necessary.

6. Place ¾ cup of couscous or other grain (if using) and 1 cup of the shrimp mixture in each of 4 containers.

STORAGE *Store covered containers in the refrigerator for up to 4 days.*

TIP *Thawed frozen shrimp emit a lot of moisture, which can cause your shrimp to steam rather than brown. Be sure to blot the shrimp with paper towels to eliminate as much moisture as possible before cooking.*

Per Serving: Total calories: 188; Total fat: 9g; Saturated fat: 1g; Sodium: 403mg; Carbohydrates: 9g; Fiber: 2g; Protein: 19g

Niçoise-Inspired Salad *with* Sardines

MAKES 4 SERVINGS

PREP TIME:
15 minutes

———

COOK TIME:
15 minutes

———

Sardines are one of the few whole foods that naturally contain vitamin D. These small yet nutritionally mighty fish are a staple in Mediterranean cuisine and are also rich in heart- and brain-healthy omega-3 fatty acids.

4 eggs

12 ounces baby red potatoes (about 12 potatoes)

6 ounces green beans, halved

4 cups baby spinach leaves or mixed greens

1 bunch radishes, quartered (about 1⅓ cups)

1 cup cherry tomatoes

20 kalamata or niçoise olives (about ⅓ cup)

3 (3.75-ounce) cans skinless, boneless sardines packed in olive oil, drained

8 tablespoons Dijon Red Wine Vinaigrette (page 177)

1. Place the eggs in a saucepan and cover with water. Bring the water to a boil. As soon as the water starts to boil, place a lid on the pan and turn the heat off. Set a timer for 12 minutes.

2. When the timer goes off, drain the hot water and run cold water over the eggs to cool. Peel the eggs when cool and cut in half.

3. Prick each potato a few times with a fork. Place them on a microwave-safe plate and microwave on high for 4 to 5 minutes, until the potatoes are tender. Let cool and cut in half.

4. Place green beans on a microwave-safe plate and microwave on high for 1½ to 2 minutes, until the beans are crisp-tender. Cool.

5. Place 1 egg, ½ cup of green beans, 6 potato halves, 1 cup of spinach, ⅓ cup of radishes, ¼ cup of tomatoes, 5 olives, and 3 sardines in each of 4 containers. Pour 2 tablespoons of vinaigrette into each of 4 sauce containers.

STORAGE *Store covered containers in the refrigerator for up to 4 days.*

Per Serving: Total calories: 450; Total fat: 32g; Saturated fat: 5g; Sodium: 673mg; Carbohydrates: 22g; Fiber: 5g; Protein: 21g

Broiled Herb Sole *with* Cauliflower Mashed Potatoes

MAKES 4 SERVINGS

PREP TIME:
10 minutes

—

COOK TIME:
16 minutes

—

I love mashing other veggies with potatoes to increase veggie variety. While this does make the dish lower in carbs, don't be scared of potatoes! They are part of the Mediterranean diet and contain many nutrients such as vitamin C, B$_6$, and fiber, making them a perfect pairing with broiled fish.

FOR THE CAULIFLOWER MASHED POTATOES

12 ounces cauliflower florets, cut into 1-inch pieces

1 (12-ounce) Yukon Gold potato, cut into ¾-inch pieces (do not peel)

2 tablespoons olive oil

¼ teaspoon kosher salt

FOR THE SOLE

2 teaspoons olive oil, plus more to grease the pan

3 tablespoons chopped parsley

3 tablespoons chopped fresh dill

1 tablespoon freshly squeezed lemon juice

½ teaspoon chopped garlic

1¼ pounds boneless, skinless sole or tilapia

¼ teaspoon kosher salt

4 lemon wedges, for serving

TO MAKE THE CAULIFLOWER MASHED POTATOES

1. Pour enough water into a saucepan that it reaches ½ inch up the side of the pan. Turn the heat to high and bring the water to a boil. Add the cauliflower and potatoes, and cover the pan. Steam for 10 minutes or until the veggies are very tender.

2. Drain the vegetables if water remains in the pan. Transfer the veggies to a large bowl and add the olive oil and salt. Taste and add an additional pinch of salt if you need it.

3. Once the veggies have cooled, scoop ¾ cup of cauliflower mashed potatoes into each of 4 containers.

TO MAKE THE SOLE

4. Preheat the oven to the high broiler setting. Line a sheet pan with foil and lightly grease the pan with oil or cooking spray.

5. Mix the oil, parsley, dill, lemon juice, and garlic in a small bowl. Pat the fish with paper towels to remove excess moisture and place on the lined sheet pan. Sprinkle the salt over the fish, then spread the herb mixture over the fish. Broil for about 6 minutes or until the fish is flaky. If your fish is very thin, broil for 5 minutes.

6. When everything has cooled, place one quarter of the fish in each of the 4 cauliflower containers. Serve with lemon wedges.

STORAGE *Store covered containers in the refrigerator for up to 4 days.*

TIP *If you don't want a watery mess on your sheet pan when you broil the fish, be sure your fish is dry before cooking. If you thawed frozen fish, you may even want to wrap it in clean dish towels to remove as much moisture as possible.*

Per Serving: Total calories: 291; Total fat: 11g; Saturated fat: 1g; Sodium: 423mg; Carbohydrates: 20g; Fiber: 2g; Protein: 29g

Lentil *and* Roasted Carrot Salad *with* Herbs *and* Feta

MAKES 4 SERVINGS

PREP TIME:
15 minutes

COOK TIME:
25 minutes

Earthy lentils, salty feta cheese, bright herbs and lemon, and sweet roasted carrots make for a delicious meat-free meal. When buying baby carrots, don't buy thin ones labeled "petite," because you want nice-size chunks to bite into. Feel free to omit the feta if you'd like to make the dish vegan.

¾ cup brown or green lentils

3 cups water

1 pound baby carrots, halved on the diagonal

2 teaspoons olive oil, plus 2 tablespoons

½ teaspoon kosher salt, divided

1 teaspoon garlic powder

1 cup packed parsley leaves, chopped

½ cup packed cilantro leaves, chopped

¼ cup packed mint leaves, chopped

½ teaspoon grated lemon zest

4 teaspoons freshly squeezed lemon juice

¼ cup crumbled feta cheese

1. Preheat the oven to 400°F. Line a sheet pan with a silicone baking mat or parchment paper.

2. Place the lentils and water in a medium saucepan and turn the heat to high. As soon as the water comes to a boil, turn the heat to low and simmer until the lentils are firm yet tender, 10 to 20 minutes (see tip on page 155). Drain and cool.

3. While the lentils are cooking, place the carrots on the sheet pan and toss with 2 teaspoons of oil, ¼ teaspoon of salt, and the garlic powder. Roast the carrots in the oven until firm yet tender, about 20 to 25 minutes. Cool when done.

4. In a large bowl, mix the cooled lentils, carrots, parsley, cilantro, mint, lemon zest, lemon juice, feta, the remaining 2 tablespoons of oil, and the remaining ¼ teaspoon of salt. Add more lemon juice and/or salt to taste if needed.

5. Place 1¼ cups of the mixture in each of 4 containers.

STORAGE   *Store covered containers in the refrigerator for up to 5 days.*

TIP   *The cooking time of lentils can vary depending on variety and age. If the lentils are very old, they may take longer than expected, with cooking times of 20 or even 30 minutes. However, start checking after 10 minutes. If they don't seem done, keep simmering, but keep a close eye on them. Cooked lentils should be firm yet tender and not mushy.*

Per Serving: Total calories: 270; Total fat: 12g; Saturated fat: 3g; Sodium: 492mg; Carbohydrates: 31g; Fiber: 13g; Protein: 12g

Quinoa Bruschetta Salad

**MAKES
5 SERVINGS**

PREP TIME:
15 minutes

———

COOK TIME:
15 minutes

———

Quinoa salads are great options for meal prep because they're sturdy enough to hold up throughout the week yet don't completely absorb all the dressing, which helps the grains remain moist and flavorful. This recipe is also a great meatless dish to round out a picnic or barbecue.

2 cups water

1 cup uncooked quinoa

1 (10-ounce) container cherry tomatoes, quartered

1 teaspoon chopped garlic

1¼ cups thinly sliced scallions, white and green parts (1 small bunch)

1 (8-ounce) container fresh whole-milk mozzarella balls (ciliegine), quartered

2 tablespoons balsamic vinegar

2 tablespoons olive oil

½ teaspoon kosher salt

½ cup fresh basil leaves, chiffonaded (cut into strips)

1. Place the water and quinoa in a saucepan and bring to a boil. Cover, turn the heat to low, and simmer for 15 minutes.

2. While the quinoa is cooking, place the tomatoes, garlic, scallions, mozzarella, vinegar, and oil in a large mixing bowl. Stir to combine.

3. Once the quinoa is cool, add it to the tomato mixture along with the salt and basil. Mix to combine.

4. Place 1⅓ cups of the mixture in each of 5 containers and refrigerate. Serve at room temperature.

STORAGE *Store covered containers in the refrigerator for up to 5 days.*

TIP *Cheese typically contains a lot of sodium; however, fresh mozzarella does not. With only 65mg per ounce, it's a great option if you love cheese but need to live a lower-sodium lifestyle.*

Per Serving: Total calories: 323; Total fat: 16g; Saturated fat: 6g; Sodium: 317mg; Carbohydrates: 30g; Fiber: 4g; Protein: 14g

Syrian Spiced Lentil, Barley, *and* Vegetable Soup

MAKES 5 SERVINGS

PREP TIME:
10 minutes

———

COOK TIME:
40 minutes

———

One of the best things about homemade soups is that their flavors continue to develop as they sit in the refrigerator. This soup is inspired by spices used in traditional Syrian lentil soups, such as fragrant cumin, coriander, and cinnamon.

1 tablespoon olive oil

1 small onion, chopped (about 2 cups)

2 medium carrots, peeled and chopped (about 1 cup)

1 celery stalk, chopped (about ½ cup)

1 teaspoon chopped garlic

1 teaspoon ground cumin

1 teaspoon ground coriander

1 teaspoon turmeric

⅛ teaspoon ground cinnamon

2 tablespoons tomato paste

¾ cup green lentils

¾ cup pearled barley

8 cups water

¾ teaspoon kosher salt

1 (5-ounce) package baby spinach leaves

2 teaspoons red wine vinegar

1. Heat the oil in a soup pot on medium-high heat. When the oil is shimmering, add the onion, carrots, celery, and garlic and sauté for 8 minutes. Add the cumin, coriander, turmeric, cinnamon, and tomato paste and cook for 2 more minutes, stirring frequently.

2. Add the lentils, barley, water, and salt to the pot and bring to a boil. Turn the heat to low and simmer for 25 minutes. Add the spinach and continue to simmer for 5 more minutes.

3. Add the vinegar and adjust the seasoning if needed.

4. Spoon 2 cups of soup into each of 5 containers.

STORAGE *Store covered containers in the refrigerator for up to 5 days.*

Per Serving: Total calories: 273; Total fat: 4g; Saturated fat: 1g; Sodium: 459mg; Carbohydrates: 50g; Fiber: 16g; Protein: 12g

Smoky Chickpea, Chard, *and* Butternut Squash Soup

MAKES 8 SERVINGS

PREP TIME:
15 minutes

———

COOK TIME:
35 minutes

———

Bacon and smoked paprika add a double punch of smokiness to this loaded veggie and chickpea soup. Chard is one of my favorite no-waste veggies, because you can eat both the leaves and the stems.

2 slices bacon (about 1 ounce), chopped

1 cup chopped onion

1 teaspoon chopped garlic

1 teaspoon smoked paprika

½ teaspoon kosher salt

2 teaspoons fresh thyme leaves, roughly chopped

1½ pounds butternut squash, peeled, seeded, and cut into 1-inch cubes

1 large bunch chard, stems and leaves chopped

2 (15.5-oz) cans low-sodium chickpeas, drained and rinsed

32 ounces low-sodium chicken broth

1 tablespoon freshly squeezed lemon juice

8 teaspoons grated Parmesan or Pecorino Romano cheese for garnish

1. Place a soup pot, at least 4½ quarts in size, on the stove over medium heat. Add the chopped bacon and cook until the fat has rendered and the bacon is crisp. Remove the bacon pieces to a plate.

2. Add the chopped onion and garlic to the same pot. Sauté in the bacon fat until the onion is soft, about 5 minutes. Add the paprika, salt, and thyme. Stir to coat the onion well. Add the squash, chard, chickpeas, and broth to the pot.

3. Turn the heat to high, bring the soup to a boil, then turn the heat down to low and simmer until the squash is tender, about 20 minutes.

4. Add the lemon juice. If necessary, add another pinch of salt to taste.

5. Place 2 cups of cooled soup in each of 4 containers and top each serving with 2 teaspoons of cheese. Store the remaining 4 servings in the freezer to eat later.

STORAGE *Store covered containers in the refrigerator for up to 5 days. If frozen, soup will last 4 months.*

TIP *To make bacon easier to cut into pieces, place it in the freezer 45 minutes before you need to slice it.*

Per Serving: Total calories: 194; Total fat: 2g; Saturated fat: 1g; Sodium: 530mg; Carbohydrates: 34g; Fiber: 11g; Protein: 12g

Whole-Wheat Pasta *with* Roasted Red Pepper Sauce *and* Fresh Mozzarella

MAKES 4 SERVINGS

PREP TIME:
15 minutes

———

COOK TIME:
40 minutes

———

Red bell pepper fun fact: They have more vitamin C than oranges! The fresh mozzarella and basil really balance out the smoky pepper sauce. If you're short on time or don't want to turn on the oven, you can make the sauce by using jarred roasted peppers and omitting the tomatoes.

3 large red bell peppers, seeds removed and cut in half

1 (10-ounce) container cherry tomatoes

2 teaspoons olive oil, plus 2 tablespoons

8 ounces whole-wheat penne or rotini

1 tablespoon plus 1 teaspoon apple cider vinegar

1 teaspoon chopped garlic

1½ teaspoons smoked paprika

¼ teaspoon kosher salt

½ cup packed fresh basil leaves, chopped

1 (8-ounce) container fresh whole-milk mozzarella balls (ciliegine), quartered

1. Preheat the oven to 400°F and line a sheet pan with a silicone baking mat or parchment paper.

2. Place the peppers and tomatoes on the pan and toss with 2 teaspoons of oil. Roast for 40 minutes.

3. While the peppers and tomatoes are roasting, cook the pasta according to the instructions on the box. Drain and place the pasta in a large mixing bowl.

4. When the peppers are cool enough to handle, peel the skin and discard. It's okay if you can't remove all the skin. Place the roasted peppers, vinegar, garlic, paprika, and salt and the remaining 2 tablespoons of oil in a blender and blend until smooth.

5. Add the pepper sauce, whole roasted tomatoes, basil, and mozzarella to the pasta and stir to combine.

6. Place a heaping 2 cups of pasta and sauce in each of 4 containers.

STORAGE *Store covered containers in the refrigerator for up to 5 days.*

TIP *When measuring dried pasta, it's helpful to know that 2 ounces of uncooked pasta equals ⅔ cup of penne, ½ cup of rotini, or ¾ cup of rigatoni.*

Per Serving: Total calories: 463; Total fat: 20g; Saturated fat: 7g; Sodium: 260mg; Carbohydrates: 54g; Fiber: 9g; Protein: 18g

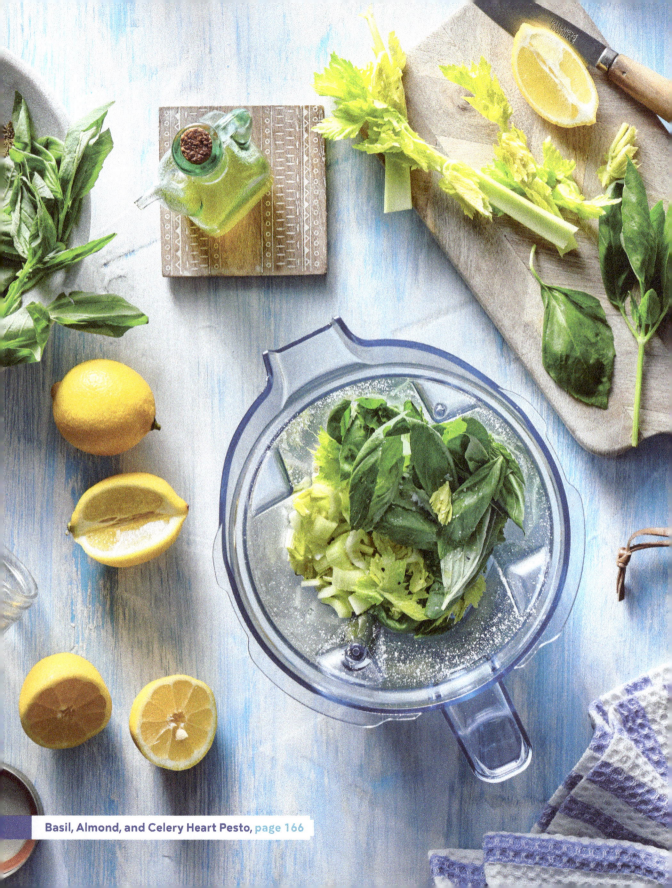

Basil, Almond, and Celery Heart Pesto, page 166

CHAPTER 11

Dips, Dressings, _and_ Sauces

Spanish Romesco Sauce

MAKES 1⅔ CUPS

PREP TIME:
10 minutes

——

COOK TIME:
10 minutes

——

Spanish romesco is delicious on a variety of foods, including chicken, fish, shrimp, veggies, roasted potatoes, and grilled bread. This recipe cuts down the prep time by using jarred peppers and canned fire-roasted tomatoes.

½ cup raw, unsalted almonds

4 medium garlic cloves (do not peel)

1 (12-ounce) jar of roasted red peppers, drained

½ cup canned diced fire-roasted tomatoes, drained

1 teaspoon smoked paprika

½ teaspoon kosher salt

Pinch cayenne pepper

2 teaspoons red wine vinegar

2 tablespoons olive oil

1. Preheat the oven to 350°F.
2. Place the almonds and garlic cloves on a sheet pan and toast in the oven for 10 minutes. Remove from the oven and peel the garlic when cool enough to handle.
3. Place the almonds in the bowl of a food processor. Process the almonds until they resemble coarse sand, 30 to 45 seconds. Add the garlic, peppers, tomatoes, paprika, salt, and cayenne. Blend until smooth.
4. Once the mixture is smooth, add the vinegar and oil and blend until well combined. Taste and add more vinegar or salt if needed.
5. Scoop the romesco sauce into a container and refrigerate.

STORAGE *Store the covered container in the refrigerator for up to 7 days.*

TIP *Freeze the extra fire-roasted tomatoes. They'll last for about 3 months in the freezer.*

Per Serving (⅓ cup): Total calories: 158; Total fat: 13g; Saturated fat: 1g; Sodium: 292mg; Carbohydrates: 10g; Fiber: 3g; Protein: 4g

Garlic Yogurt Sauce

MAKES 1 CUP

PREP TIME:
5 minutes
____

If you've never tried a savory yogurt dish before, this recipe will be a revelation! You can introduce lots of different flavors to switch up this base recipe.

1 cup low-fat (2%) plain Greek yogurt

½ teaspoon garlic powder

1 tablespoon freshly squeezed lemon juice

1 tablespoon olive oil

¼ teaspoon kosher salt

1. Mix all the ingredients in a medium bowl until well combined.

2. Spoon the yogurt sauce into a container and refrigerate.

STORAGE *Store the covered container in the refrigerator for up to 7 days.*

TIP *You can use nonfat, low-fat, or whole-milk yogurt for this recipe.*

Per Serving (¼ cup): Total calories: 75; Total fat: 5g; Saturated fat: 1g; Sodium: 173mg; Carbohydrates: 3g; Fiber: 0g; Protein: 6g.

Basil, Almond, _and_ Celery Heart Pesto

MAKES 1 CUP

PREP TIME:
10 minutes
___

My husband loves celery sticks but never eats the celery heart! My solution was to add the celery heart to the pesto to avoid throwing it in the trash. Celery is packed with vitamins and minerals, including vitamin K, folate, and potassium. This pesto is great as a sandwich spread or to top proteins like grilled chicken and fish.

½ cup raw, unsalted almonds

3 cups fresh basil leaves, (about 1½ ounces)

½ cup chopped celery hearts with leaves

¼ teaspoon kosher salt

1 tablespoon freshly squeezed lemon juice

¼ cup olive oil

3 tablespoons water

1. Place the almonds in the bowl of a food processor and process until they look like coarse sand.
2. Add the basil, celery hearts, salt, lemon juice, oil and water and process until smooth. The sauce will be somewhat thick. If you would like a thinner sauce, add more water, oil, or lemon juice, depending on your taste preference.
3. Scoop the pesto into a container and refrigerate.

STORAGE _Store the covered container in the refrigerator for up to 2 weeks. Pesto may be frozen for up to 6 months._

TIP _If you don't own a food processor, you can also make pesto in the blender. Just make sure you put the heavier items into the blender first. If your blender isn't the high-speed variety, you may also have some larger chunks of nuts._

Per Serving (¼ cup): Total calories: 231; Total fat: 22g; Saturated fat: 3g; Sodium: 178mg; Carbohydrates: 6g; Fiber: 3g; Protein: 4g

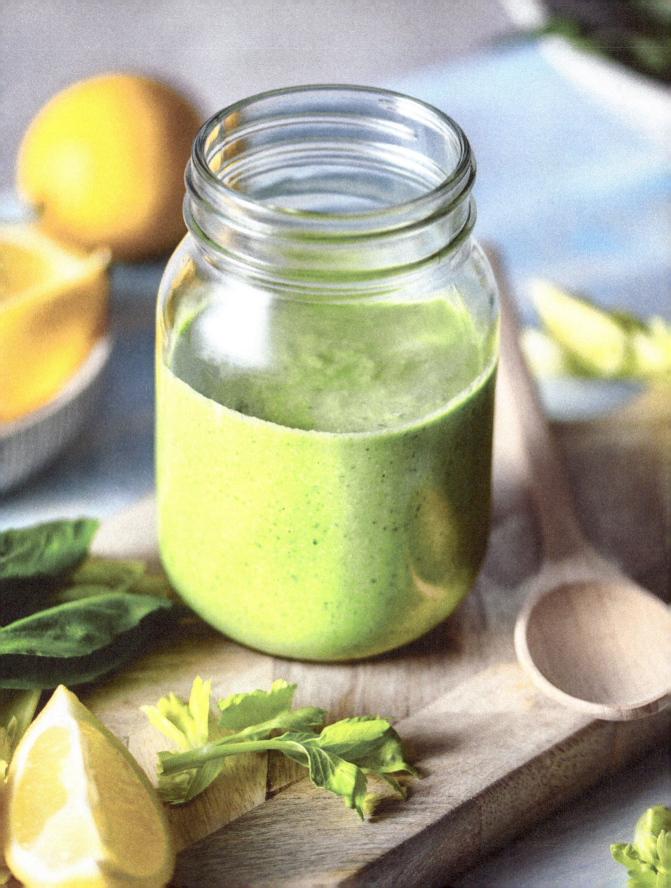

Chermoula Sauce

MAKES 1 CUP

PREP TIME:
10 minutes

Chermoula is a popular North African herb sauce that contains fresh herbs and olive oil, along with flavorful spices such as cumin and paprika. In addition to using it as a sauce to top proteins and veggies, you can also use it as a marinade.

1 cup packed parsley leaves

1 cup cilantro leaves

½ cup mint leaves

1 teaspoon chopped garlic

½ teaspoon ground cumin

½ teaspoon ground coriander

½ teaspoon smoked paprika

⅛ teaspoon cayenne pepper

⅛ teaspoon kosher salt

3 tablespoons freshly squeezed lemon juice

3 tablespoons water

½ cup extra-virgin olive oil

1. Place all the ingredients in a blender or food processor and blend until smooth.
2. Pour the chermoula into a container and refrigerate.

STORAGE _Store the covered container in the refrigerator for up to 5 days._

TIP _If you don't want to use a blender or food processor, you can make a chunkier sauce by hand-chopping the herbs and mixing them with the garlic, spices, salt, lemon juice, and oil. Add water to thin if necessary._

Per Serving (¼ cup): Total calories: 257; Total fat: 27g; Saturated fat: 4g; Sodium: 96mg; Carbohydrates: 4g; Fiber: 2g; Protein: 1g

White Bean *and* Mushroom Dip

MAKES 3 CUPS

PREP TIME:
10 minutes

———

COOK TIME:
8 minutes

———

Beans offer one of the most affordable sources of protein and fiber. Their creaminess pairs perfectly with earthy mushrooms, which, when exposed to UV light, are the only plant food that contains vitamin D! If your store sells shiitake mushrooms, add some of those for a more intense mushroom flavor.

2 teaspoons olive oil, plus 2 tablespoons

8 ounces button or cremini mushrooms, sliced

1 teaspoon chopped garlic

1 tablespoon fresh thyme leaves

2 (15.5-ounce) cans cannellini beans, drained and rinsed

2 tablespoons plus 1 teaspoon freshly squeezed lemon juice

½ teaspoon kosher salt

1. Heat 2 teaspoons of oil in a 12-inch skillet over medium-high heat. Once the oil is shimmering, add the mushrooms and sauté for 6 minutes. Add the garlic and thyme and continue cooking for 2 minutes.

2. While the mushrooms are cooking, place the beans and lemon juice, the remaining 2 tablespoons of oil, and the salt in the bowl of a food processor. Add the mushrooms as soon as they are done cooking and blend everything until smooth. Scrape down the sides of the bowl if necessary and continue to process until smooth.

3. Taste and adjust the seasoning with lemon juice or salt if needed.

4. Scoop the dip into a container and refrigerate.

STORAGE *Store the covered container in the refrigerator for up to 5 days. Dip can be frozen for up to 3 months.*

TIP *Try using other beans, such as pinto, black, or kidney beans, or even lentils to make dips.*

Per Serving (½ cup): Total calories: 192; Total fat: 6g; Saturated fat: 1g; Sodium: 197mg; Carbohydrates: 25g; Fiber: 7g; Protein: 9g

Roasted Eggplant Dip (Baba Ghanoush)

**MAKES
2 CUPS**

PREP TIME:
10 minutes

———

COOK TIME:
45 minutes

———

Baba ghanoush is a popular dip in many countries, including Lebanon, Israel, and Syria, and you don't need a blender or food processor to make it. The eggplant gets so tender that you can easily mash it with a fork.

2 eggplants (close to 1 pound each)

1 teaspoon chopped garlic

3 tablespoons unsalted tahini

¼ cup freshly squeezed lemon juice

1 tablespoon olive oil

½ teaspoon kosher salt

1. Preheat the oven to 450°F and line a sheet pan with a silicone baking mat or parchment paper.

2. Prick the eggplants in many places with a fork, place on the sheet pan, and roast in the oven until extremely soft, about 45 minutes. The eggplants should look like they are deflating.

3. When the eggplants are cool, cut them open and scoop the flesh into a large bowl. You may need to use your hands to pull the flesh away from the skin. Discard the skin. Mash the flesh very well with a fork.

4. Add the garlic, tahini, lemon juice, oil, and salt. Taste and adjust the seasoning with additional lemon juice, salt, or tahini if needed.

5. Scoop the dip into a container and refrigerate.

STORAGE *Store the covered container in the refrigerator for up to 5 days.*

TIP *One juicy lemon usually contains ¼ cup of juice. Buy more than 1 lemon at the store, just in case you need to add additional lemon juice to suit your taste buds.*

Per Serving (¼ cup): Total calories: 87; Total fat: 5g; Saturated fat: 1g; Sodium: 156mg; Carbohydrates: 10g; Fiber: 4g; Protein: 2g

Hummus

PREP TIME:
5 minutes

———

We can't talk about the Mediterranean diet without mentioning hummus. Even just a few tablespoons contain a nice amount of fiber, protein, and healthy fats, as well as a wide range of vitamins and minerals. Not only is it fabulous as a veggie dip, but also it's great as a sandwich or wrap spread.

**1 (15-ounce) can
low-sodium chickpeas,
drained and rinsed**

¼ cup unsalted tahini

½ teaspoon chopped garlic

**¼ cup freshly squeezed
lemon juice**

¼ teaspoon kosher salt

3 tablespoons olive oil

3 tablespoons cold water

1. Place all the ingredients in a food processor or blender and blend until smooth.
2. Taste and adjust the seasonings if needed.
3. Scoop the hummus into a container and refrigerate.

STORAGE *Store the covered container in the refrigerator for up to 5 days.*

TIP *Hummus is a great vehicle for using up fresh herbs you may have in the refrigerator. Try adding parsley or cilantro. You can also add spices, such as paprika or cumin.*

Per Serving (¼ cup): Total calories: 192; Total fat: 13g; Saturated fat: 2g; Sodium: 109mg; Carbohydrates: 16g; Fiber: 5g; Protein: 5g

Green Olive *and* Spinach Tapenade

**MAKES
1½ CUPS**

PREP TIME:
10 minutes

I could eat this tapenade on top of everything! The saltiness from the olives, herbal flavors from the basil and oregano, and acid from the vinegar really balance well. It's delicious on top of chicken, meat, or fish, or pair it with the baked tofu from Tofu and Vegetable Provençal (page 77).

1 cup pimento-stuffed green olives, drained

3 packed cups baby spinach

1 teaspoon chopped garlic

½ teaspoon dried oregano

⅓ cup packed fresh basil

2 tablespoons olive oil

2 teaspoons red wine vinegar

1. Place all the ingredients in the bowl of a food processor and pulse until the mixture looks finely chopped but not puréed.
2. Scoop the tapenade into a container and refrigerate.

STORAGE *Store the covered container in the refrigerator for up to 5 days.*

TIP *Feel free to substitute black olives or use a mixture of black and green olives.*

Per Serving (¼ cup): Total calories: 80; Total fat: 8g; Saturated fat: 1g; Sodium: 436mg; Carbohydrates: 1g; Fiber: 1g; Protein: 1g

Artichoke-Olive Compote

**MAKES
1⅓ CUPS**

PREP TIME:
5 minutes

___

This compote is the perfect topping for grilled chicken, steak, fish, and vegetables. It's also great mixed into a simply prepared whole grain like bulgur, brown rice, or farro. Feel free to use kalamata or oil-cured black olives, or even a mix of black and green olives if you prefer.

1 (6-ounce) jar marinated artichoke hearts, chopped

⅓ cup chopped pitted green olives (8 to 9 olives)

3 tablespoons chopped fresh basil

½ teaspoon freshly squeezed lemon juice

2 teaspoons olive oil

1. Place all the ingredients in a medium mixing bowl and stir to combine.

2. Place the compote in a container and refrigerate.

STORAGE *Store the covered container in the refrigerator for up to 7 days.*

TIP *If you don't want to buy a whole jar of olives, buy a small amount from your supermarket's salad bar. Oftentimes you'll find a variety of olives that can be mixed and matched and purchased by weight.*

___

Per Serving (⅓ cup): Total calories: 84; Total fat: 7g; Saturated fat: 1g; Sodium: 350mg; Carbohydrates: 5g; Fiber: <1g; Protein: <1g

Chunky Roasted Cherry Tomato _and_ Basil Sauce

MAKES
1⅓ CUPS

PREP TIME:
10 minutes

___

COOK TIME:
40 minutes

___

Roasting brings the sweetness of cherry tomatoes to a whole new level! This sauce makes a great topping for fish or chicken, especially Mediterranean-Style Pesto Chicken (page 131). You can also mix this with Garlic Yogurt Sauce (page 165) for a rich and creamy sauce.

2 pints cherry tomatoes (20 ounces total)

2 teaspoons olive oil, plus 3 tablespoons

¼ teaspoon kosher salt

½ teaspoon chopped garlic

¼ cup fresh basil leaves

1. Preheat the oven to 350°F. Line a sheet pan with a silicone baking mat or parchment paper.
2. Place the tomatoes on the lined sheet pan and toss with 2 teaspoons of oil. Roast for 40 minutes, shaking the pan halfway through.
3. While the tomatoes are still warm, place them in a medium mixing bowl and add the salt, the garlic, and the remaining 3 tablespoons of oil. Mash the tomatoes with the back of a fork. Stir in the fresh basil.
4. Scoop the sauce into a container and refrigerate.

STORAGE _Store the covered container in the refrigerator for up to 5 days._

TIP _Try adding a pinch of red chili flakes if you like heat._

Per Serving (⅓ cup): Total calories: 141; Total fat: 13g; Saturated fat: 2g; Sodium: 158mg; Carbohydrates: 7g; Fiber: 2g; Protein: 1g

Tzatziki Sauce

**MAKES
2½ CUPS**

PREP TIME:
15 minutes

———

Tzatziki is a classic Greek yogurt sauce made with refreshing cucumber, lemon, and dill. Some versions also contain fresh mint, which I've included in my recipe. Use as a dip with crackers and veggies, as a sauce for grilled meats, or straight up as a snack.

1 English cucumber

2 cups low-fat (2%) plain Greek yogurt

1 tablespoon olive oil

2 teaspoons freshly squeezed lemon juice

½ teaspoon chopped garlic

½ teaspoon kosher salt

⅛ teaspoon freshly ground black pepper

2 tablespoons chopped fresh dill

2 tablespoons chopped fresh mint

1. Place a sieve over a medium bowl. Grate the cucumber, with the skin, over the sieve. Press the grated cucumber into the sieve with the flat surface of a spatula to press as much liquid out as possible.

2. In a separate medium bowl, place the yogurt, oil, lemon juice, garlic, salt, pepper, dill, and mint and stir to combine.

3. Press on the cucumber one last time, then add it to the yogurt mixture. Stir to combine. Taste and add more salt and lemon juice if necessary.

4. Scoop the sauce into a container and refrigerate.

STORAGE *Store the covered container in the refrigerator for up to 5 days.*

TIP *If you don't want to grate the cucumber, you can also finely chop it or pulse it in a food processor.*

Per Serving (¼ cup): Total calories: 51; Total fat: 2g; Saturated fat: 1g; Sodium: 137mg; Carbohydrates: 3g; Fiber: <1g; Protein: 5g

Raspberry Red Wine Sauce

MAKES ABOUT 1 CUP

PREP TIME:
5 minutes

——

COOK TIME:
20 minutes

——

Red wine and raspberries are a flavor match made in heaven, and both are rich in antioxidants, including resveratrol, which has been linked to reducing the risk of cancer and heart disease. Try using a red wine that contains notes of raspberry, such as red zinfandel, cabernet sauvignon, pinot noir, or tempranillo.

2 teaspoons olive oil

2 tablespoons finely chopped shallot

1½ cups frozen raspberries

1 cup dry, fruity red wine

1 teaspoon thyme leaves, roughly chopped

1 teaspoon honey

¼ teaspoon kosher salt

½ teaspoon unsweetened cocoa powder

1. In a 10-inch skillet, heat the oil over medium heat. Add the shallot and cook until soft, about 2 minutes.

2. Add the raspberries, wine, thyme, and honey and cook on medium heat until reduced, about 15 minutes. Stir in the salt and cocoa powder.

3. Transfer the sauce to a blender and blend until smooth. Depending on how much you can scrape out of your blender, this recipe makes ¾ to 1 cup of sauce.

4. Scoop the sauce into a container and refrigerate.

STORAGE *Store the covered container in the refrigerator for up to 7 days.*

TIP *When blending hot liquids, use caution to avoid burning yourself. Make sure the lid is on tightly and covered with a towel when blending, and open the blender very slowly when done.*

Per Serving (¼ cup): Total calories: 107; Total fat: 3g; Saturated fat: <1g; Sodium: 148mg; Carbohydrates: 1g; Fiber: 4g; Protein: 1g

Dijon Red Wine Vinaigrette

MAKES ½ CUP

PREP TIME:
5 minutes

——

Homemade dressing is so easy to make. It's healthier than store-bought versions and contains much less sodium. The Dijon mustard helps bind the dressing together and create a creamy consistency.

2 teaspoons Dijon mustard

3 tablespoons red wine vinegar

1 tablespoon water

¼ teaspoon dried oregano

¼ teaspoon chopped garlic

⅛ teaspoon kosher salt

¼ cup olive oil

1. Place the mustard, vinegar, water, oregano, garlic, and salt in a small bowl and whisk to combine.

2. Whisk in the oil, pouring it into the mustard-vinegar mixture in a thin steam.

3. Pour the vinaigrette into a container and refrigerate.

STORAGE *Store the covered container in the refrigerator for up to 2 weeks. Allow the vinaigrette to come to room temperature and shake before serving.*

TIP *Don't want to chop garlic and get your hands stinky? Use chopped garlic found in the produce section. In fact, many restaurants use this option, as well! This dressing recipe can easily be doubled if you'd like to have it on hand in greater quantity.*

Per Serving (2 tablespoons): Total calories: 123; Total fat: 14g; Saturated fat: 2g; Sodium: 133mg; Carbohydrates: 0g; Fiber: 0g; Protein: 0g

Honey-Lemon Vinaigrette

MAKES
½ CUP

PREP TIME:
5 minutes

———

Vinaigrettes are super easy to make. They contain so much flavor, and they can do a lot more than just dress lettuce-based salads. Add them to slaws and grains, or drizzle them over grilled or roasted veggies, chicken, fish, and meat.

¼ cup freshly squeezed lemon juice

1 teaspoon honey

2 teaspoons Dijon mustard

⅛ teaspoon kosher salt

¼ cup olive oil

1. Place the lemon juice, honey, mustard, and salt in a small bowl and whisk to combine.

2. Whisk in the oil, pouring it into the bowl in a thin steam.

3. Pour the vinaigrette into a container and refrigerate.

STORAGE *Store the covered container in the refrigerator for up to 2 weeks. Allow the vinaigrette to come to room temperature and shake before serving.*

TIP *You can also make a vinaigrette in a mason jar by pouring all the ingredients into the jar and shaking until well combined.*

Per Serving (2 tablespoons): Total calories: 131; Total fat: 14g; Saturated fat: 2g; Sodium: 133mg; Carbohydrates: 3g; Fiber: <1g; Protein: <1g

Pomegranate Vinaigrette

**MAKES
½ CUP**

PREP TIME:
5 minutes

——

Pomegranate is one of the healthiest fruits around and may be especially beneficial for brain and heart health. Its anti-inflammatory effects come from a class of antioxidants called polyphenols. Packed with nutrients, it is also sweet, slightly tart, and delicious!

⅓ cup pomegranate juice

1 teaspoon Dijon mustard

1 tablespoon apple cider vinegar

½ teaspoon dried mint

2 tablespoons plus 2 teaspoons olive oil

1. Place the pomegranate juice, mustard, vinegar, and mint in a small bowl and whisk to combine.

2. Whisk in the oil, pouring it into the bowl in a thin steam.

3. Pour the vinaigrette into a container and refrigerate.

STORAGE *Store the covered container in the refrigerator for up to 2 weeks. Bring the vinaigrette to room temperature and shake before serving.*

TIP *You don't need to buy a big bottle of pomegranate juice for this recipe. Many supermarkets sell convenient 16-fluid-ounce bottles in the produce section. Use the leftovers for smoothies!*

Per Serving (2 tablespoons): Total calories: 94; Total fat: 10g; Saturated fat: 2g; Sodium: 30mg; Carbohydrates: 3g; Fiber: 0g; Protein: 0g

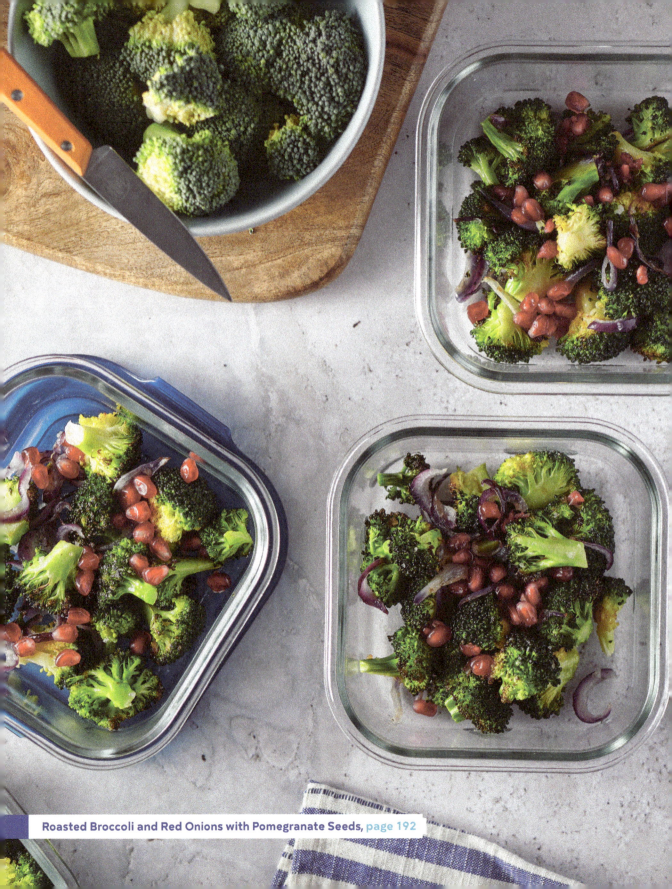

Roasted Broccoli and Red Onions with Pomegranate Seeds, page 192

Sides, Snacks, _and_ Sweets

DAIRY-FREE • GLUTEN-FREE • VEGAN

Candied Maple-Cinnamon Walnuts

**MAKES
4 SERVINGS**

PREP TIME:
5 minutes

———

COOK TIME:
15 minutes

———

Some candied walnuts are deep-fried and tossed in a ton of powdered sugar. So not healthy! This baked version is still sweet and tasty but much healthier.

1 cup walnut halves

**½ teaspoon
ground cinnamon**

**2 tablespoons pure
maple syrup**

1. Preheat the oven to 325°F. Line a baking sheet with a silicone baking mat or parchment paper.

2. In a small bowl, mix the walnuts, cinnamon, and maple syrup until the walnuts are coated.

3. Pour the nuts onto the baking sheet, making sure to scrape out all the maple syrup. Bake for 15 minutes. Allow the nuts to cool completely.

4. Place ¼ cup of nuts in each of 4 containers or resealable sandwich bags.

STORAGE *Store covered containers at room temperature for up to 7 days.*

TIP *If you use walnut pieces instead of halves, the baking time may be less. Pecans would also work well with this recipe.*

Per Serving: Total calories: 190; Total fat: 17g; Saturated fat: 2g; Sodium: 2mg; Carbohydrates: 10g; Fiber: 2g; Protein: 4g

Cardamom Mascarpone *with* Strawberries

PREP TIME:
10 minutes

_____

This whipped spiced mascarpone tastes like a thicker, rich version of whipped cream. It's one of the easiest desserts you can make and will definitely satisfy your sweet tooth.

1 (8-ounce) container mascarpone cheese

2 teaspoons honey

¼ teaspoon ground cardamom

2 tablespoons milk

1 pound strawberries (should be 24 strawberries in the pack)

1. Combine the mascarpone, honey, cardamom, and milk in a medium mixing bowl.
2. Mix the ingredients with a spoon until super creamy, about 30 seconds.
3. Place 6 strawberries and 2 tablespoons of the mascarpone mixture in each of 4 containers.

STORAGE *Store covered containers in the refrigerator for up to 5 days.*

TIP *You can use any milk you have on hand, including cow's milk, almond milk, or even coconut milk. Also, if you don't have cardamom, give cinnamon a try.*

Per Serving: Total calories: 289; Total fat: 25g; Saturated fat: 10g; Sodium: 26mg; Carbohydrates: 11g; Fiber: 3g; Protein: 1g

Mocha-Nut Stuffed Dates

**MAKES
5 SERVINGS**

PREP TIME:
10 minutes

___

Dates are nature's candy! You may see Medjool dates and another variety called Deglet Noor. Medjool are typically larger and softer, which makes them great for stuffing with fillings. Visually inspect the dates to make sure they aren't dry and cracked.

2 tablespoons creamy, unsweetened, unsalted almond butter

1 teaspoon unsweetened cocoa powder

3 tablespoons walnut pieces

2 tablespoons water

¼ teaspoon honey

¾ teaspoon instant espresso powder

10 Medjool dates, pitted

1. In a small bowl, combine the almond butter, cocoa powder, and walnut pieces.
2. Place the water in a small microwaveable mug and heat on high for 30 seconds. Add the honey and espresso powder to the water and stir to dissolve.
3. Add the espresso water to the cocoa bowl and combine thoroughly until a creamy, thick paste forms.
4. Stuff each pitted date with 1 teaspoon of mocha filling.
5. Place 2 dates in each of 5 small containers.

STORAGE *Store covered containers in the refrigerator for up to 5 days.*

TIP *Instant espresso powder is actually meant for baking and surprisingly not for drinking! It's often the secret ingredient many professional pastry chefs use to enhance the chocolate flavor of chocolate desserts.*

Per Serving: Total calories: 205; Total fat: 7g; Saturated fat: 1g; Sodium: 1mg; Carbohydrates: 39g; Fiber: 4g; Protein: 3g

Fruit Salad *with* Mint *and* Orange Blossom Water

**MAKES
5 SERVINGS**

PREP TIME:
10 minutes

Liven up your fruit salad with the exotic aroma of orange blossom water! This ingredient, usually found in the international aisle of the supermarket, has a floral scent that transforms ordinary fruit salad into something special. If you can't find it, try adding a dash of freshly squeezed orange juice and zest.

3 cups cantaloupe, cut into 1-inch cubes

2 cups hulled and halved strawberries

½ teaspoon orange blossom water

2 tablespoons chopped fresh mint

1. In a large bowl, toss all the ingredients together.
2. Place 1 cup of fruit salad in each of 5 containers.

STORAGE *Store covered containers in the refrigerator for up to 5 days.*

TIP *Mix up your fruit based on seasonality and what looks good at the market. Mint and orange blossom will taste good with any fruit you choose.*

Per Serving: Total calories: 52; Total fat: 1g; Saturated fat: <1g; Sodium: 10mg; Carbohydrates: 12g; Fiber: 2g; Protein: 1g

Sweet *and* Spicy Green Pumpkin Seeds

**MAKES
2 CUPS**

PREP TIME:
10 minutes

———

COOK TIME:
15 minutes

———

Pepitas are green, hull-less pumpkin seeds that come from a specific type of pumpkin. They aren't the same as the seeds from your Halloween pumpkin. Rich in zinc, iron, and magnesium, pepitas are a nutrient-rich, nut-free snack.

2 cups raw green pumpkin seeds (pepitas)

1 egg white, beaten until frothy

3 tablespoons honey

1 tablespoon chili powder

¼ teaspoon cayenne pepper

1 teaspoon ground cinnamon

¼ teaspoon kosher salt

1. Preheat the oven to 350°F. Line a sheet pan with a silicone baking mat or parchment paper.

2. In a medium bowl, mix all the ingredients until the seeds are well coated. Place on the lined sheet pan in a single, even layer.

3. Bake for 15 minutes. Cool the seeds on the sheet pan, then peel clusters from the baking mat and break apart into small pieces.

4. Place ¼ cup of seeds in each of 8 small containers or resealable sandwich bags.

STORAGE *Store covered containers or resealable bags at room temperature for up to 5 days.*

TIP *If you like spicy food, add an additional ⅛ to ¼ teaspoon cayenne pepper.*

Per Serving (¼ cup): Total calories: 209; Total fat: 15g; Saturated fat: 3g; Sodium: 85mg; Carbohydrates: 11g; Fiber: 2g; Protein: 10g

Blueberry, Flax, *and* Sunflower Butter Bites

MAKES 6 SERVINGS

PREP TIME:
10 minutes,
plus
20 minutes
freezing
time

————

Many recipes for energy bites contain either almond butter or peanut butter as the binder. If you prefer a nut-free version, sunflower seed butter is the perfect substitute. Combined with the delicious flavors of blueberries and lemon zest, this snack can double as a sweet treat.

¼ cup ground flaxseed

½ cup unsweetened sunflower butter, preferably unsalted

⅓ cup dried blueberries

2 tablespoons all-fruit blueberry preserves

Zest of 1 lemon

2 tablespoons unsalted sunflower seeds

⅓ cup rolled oats

1. Mix all the ingredients in a medium mixing bowl until well combined.
2. Form 12 balls, slightly smaller than a golf ball, from the mixture and place on a plate in the freezer for about 20 minutes to firm up.
3. Place 2 bites in each of 6 containers and refrigerate.

STORAGE *Store covered containers in the refrigerator for up to 5 days. Bites may also be stored in the freezer for up to 3 months.*

TIP *When choosing fruit preserves, look at the ingredient label. Ideally, you want a product that is sweetened by fruit juice and not added granulated sugar or corn syrup. Look for the term "all-fruit" on the front of the package.*

Per Serving: Total calories: 229; Total fat: 14g; Saturated fat: 1g; Sodium: 1mg; Carbohydrates: 26g; Fiber: 3g; Protein: 7g

Pesto Deviled Eggs *with* Sun-Dried Tomatoes

MAKES 5 SERVINGS

PREP TIME:
10 minutes

COOK TIME:
15 minutes

If you're bored with the usual deviled eggs, try adding pesto and sun-dried tomatoes to liven them up, Mediterranean style. This recipe omits the typical mayonnaise and substitutes healthier plain Greek yogurt to make the filling extra creamy.

5 large eggs

3 tablespoons prepared pesto

¼ teaspoon white vinegar

2 tablespoons low-fat (2%) plain Greek yogurt

5 teaspoons sliced sun-dried tomatoes

1. Place the eggs in a saucepan and cover with water. Bring the water to a boil. As soon as the water starts to boil, place a lid on the pan and turn the heat off. Set a timer for 12 minutes.

2. When the timer goes off, drain the hot water and run cold water over the eggs to cool.

3. Peel the eggs, slice in half vertically, and scoop out the yolks. Place the yolks in a medium mixing bowl and add the pesto, vinegar, and yogurt. Mix well, until creamy.

4. Scoop about 1 tablespoon of the pesto-yolk mixture into each egg half. Top each with ½ teaspoon of sun-dried tomatoes.

5. Place 2 stuffed egg halves in each of 5 separate containers.

STORAGE *Store covered containers in the refrigerator for up to 5 days.*

TIP *For a twist, try using sun-dried tomato pesto instead of regular pesto and omitting the sliced tomatoes.*

Per Serving: Total calories: 124; Total fat: 9g; Saturated fat: 2g; Sodium: 204mg; Carbohydrates: 2g; Fiber: <1g; Protein: 8g

Antipasti Shrimp Skewers

MAKES 4 SERVINGS

PREP TIME:
10 minutes

___

I'm not sure why, but food on a stick is so much fun! It's a great way to fit many different flavors into one snack. Fresh mozzarella balls work well because their size is similar to the cherry tomatoes, making them perfect for a uniform skewer. Look on the front of the package for the word "ciliegine."

16 pitted kalamata or green olives

16 fresh mozzarella balls (ciliegine)

16 cherry tomatoes

16 medium (41 to 50 per pound) precooked peeled, deveined shrimp

8 (8-inch) wooden or metal skewers

1. Alternate 2 olives, 2 mozzarella balls, 2 cherry tomatoes, and 2 shrimp on 8 skewers.
2. Place 2 skewers in each of 4 containers.

STORAGE *Store covered containers in the refrigerator for up to 4 days.*

TIP *Try mixing up the ingredients that go on your skewers. You can use items such as prosciutto, raw summer squash and bell peppers, artichoke hearts, peppadews, and whole pepperoncini.*

Per Serving: Total calories: 108; Total fat: 6g; Saturated fat: 1g; Sodium: 328mg; Carbohydrates: 4g; Fiber: 1g; Protein: 9g

Smoked Paprika *and* Olive Oil–Marinated Carrots

PREP TIME:
10 minutes

——

COOK TIME:
5 minutes

——

Baby carrots serve more purposes than just snacking on raw or dipping into hummus. They're the perfect size for a hot vegetable side and only take 5 minutes to steam. This dish can be served warm or at room temperature.

1 (1-pound) bag baby carrots (not the petite size)

2 tablespoons olive oil

2 tablespoons red wine vinegar

¼ teaspoon garlic powder

¼ teaspoon ground cumin

¼ teaspoon smoked paprika

⅛ teaspoon red pepper flakes

¼ cup chopped parsley

¼ teaspoon kosher salt

1. Pour enough water into a saucepan to come ¼ inch up the sides. Turn the heat to high, bring the water to a boil, add the carrots, and cover with a lid. Steam the carrots for 5 minutes, until crisp tender.

2. After the carrots have cooled, mix with the oil, vinegar, garlic powder, cumin, paprika, red pepper, parsley, and salt.

3. Place ¾ cup of carrots in each of 4 containers.

STORAGE *Store covered containers in the refrigerator for up to 5 days.*

TIP *If you prefer sautéed or roasted veggies, you can also use those cooking methods for this dish. You can even swap the carrots for other veggies such as cauliflower or green beans.*

Per Serving: Total calories: 109; Total fat: 7g; Saturated fat: 1g; Sodium: 234mg; Carbohydrates: 11g; Fiber: 3g; Protein: 2g

Sautéed Kale *with* Garlic *and* Lemon

**MAKES
4 SERVINGS**

PREP TIME:
5 minutes

——

COOK TIME:
7 minutes

——

Kale is such a versatile veggie and can be used in many applications, but my favorite way to cook kale is simply to sauté it. Garlic and lemon are classic flavors that can be used with any green vegetable. Fresh, simple, easy, and delicious!

1 tablespoon olive oil

3 bunches kale, stemmed and roughly chopped

2 teaspoons chopped garlic

¼ teaspoon kosher salt

1 tablespoon freshly squeezed lemon juice

1. Heat the oil in a 12-inch skillet over medium-high heat. Once the oil is shimmering, add as much kale as will fit in the pan. You will probably only fit half the leaves into the pan at first. Mix the kale with tongs so that the leaves are coated with oil and start to wilt. As the kale wilts, keep adding more of the raw kale, continuing to use tongs to mix. Once all the kale is in the pan, add the garlic and salt and continue to cook until the kale is tender. Total cooking time from start to finish should be about 7 minutes.

2. Mix the lemon juice into the kale. Add additional salt and/or lemon juice if necessary.

3. Place 1 cup of kale in each of 4 containers and refrigerate.

STORAGE   *Store covered containers in the refrigerator for up to 5 days.*

TIP   *Three bunches of kale should equal about 1½ pounds. If you purchase precut bagged kale without the stems from the supermarket, you'll need about 15 ounces.*

Per Serving: Total calories: 85; Total fat: 1g; Saturated fat: <1g; Sodium: 214mg; Carbohydrates: 17g; Fiber: 6g; Protein: 6g

Roasted Broccoli *and* Red Onions *with* Pomegranate Seeds

MAKES 5 SERVINGS

PREP TIME:
5 minutes

———

COOK TIME:
20 minutes

———

Roasted veggies are great for meal prep, because they're so easy to make in large batches. One of the keys to getting nice brown caramelization on roasted vegetables is to avoid overcrowding the pan. If the vegetables are too close together in the pan, you end up steaming them, so use two sheet pans to make sure the veggies get great color and texture.

1 (12-ounce) package broccoli florets (about 6 cups)

1 small red onion, thinly sliced

2 tablespoons olive oil

¼ teaspoon kosher salt

1 (5.3-ounce) container pomegranate seeds (1 cup)

1. Preheat the oven to 425°F and line 2 sheet pans with silicone baking mats or parchment paper.

2. Place the broccoli and onion on the sheet pans and toss with the oil and salt. Place the pans in the oven and roast for 20 minutes.

3. After removing the pans from the oven, cool the veggies, then toss with the pomegranate seeds.

4. Place 1 cup of veggies in each of 5 containers.

STORAGE *Store covered containers in the refrigerator for up to 5 days.*

TIP *You don't need to buy a whole pomegranate to get the seeds. Pomegranate seeds are sold year-round in the produce section where the cut-up fruit and refrigerated juices are kept. If you buy a whole pomegranate, cut a slit in the fruit, fill a large bowl with water, submerge the fruit, and break it open underwater. By pulling the seeds from the skin underwater, you won't stain yourself or the kitchen counter red.*

Per Serving: Total calories: 118; Total fat: 6g; Saturated fat: 1g; Sodium: 142mg; Carbohydrates: 12g; Fiber: 4g; Protein: 2g

North African Spiced Sautéed Cabbage

MAKES 4 SERVINGS

PREP TIME:
5 minutes
——

COOK TIME:
10 minutes
——

Green cabbage is the ultimate budget-friendly vegetable! Plus, it's a cruciferous veggie that contains cancer-fighting compounds. The spice mix used in this recipe, tabil, is used in Tunisia and Algeria and has quickly become a favorite of mine. If you like spicy food, add a generous sprinkling of red chili flakes.

2 teaspoons olive oil

1 small head green cabbage (about 1½ to 2 pounds), cored and thinly sliced

1 teaspoon ground coriander

1 teaspoon garlic powder

½ teaspoon caraway seeds

½ teaspoon ground cumin

¼ teaspoon kosher salt

Pinch red chili flakes (optional—if you don't like heat, omit it)

1 teaspoon freshly squeezed lemon juice

1. Heat the oil in a 12-inch skillet over medium-high heat. Once the oil is hot, add the cabbage and cook down for 3 minutes. Add the coriander, garlic powder, caraway seeds, cumin, salt, and chili flakes (if using) and stir to combine. Continue cooking the cabbage for about 7 more minutes.

2. Stir in the lemon juice and cool.

3. Place 1 heaping cup of cabbage in each of 4 containers.

STORAGE *Store covered containers in the refrigerator for up to 5 days.*

TIP *To make slicing cabbage more manageable, cut the head of cabbage into quarters first. It's much easier to cut something when you break it down into smaller pieces.*

Per Serving: Total calories: 69; Total fat: 3g; Saturated fat: <1g; Sodium: 178mg; Carbohydrates: 11g; Fiber: 4g; Protein: 3g

Orange _and_ Cinnamon–Scented Whole-Wheat Couscous

MAKES 4 SERVINGS

PREP TIME:
5 minutes
——

COOK TIME:
10 minutes
——

Did you know that couscous is actually pasta? It's wheat flour formed into teeny-tiny balls. Many supermarkets sell whole-wheat couscous, which is the healthier option because it provides more fiber. If you can't find the whole-wheat version, use regular couscous. It's fine to include non-whole-grain options in your diet, but remember to choose whole grains on most occasions.

2 teaspoons olive oil

¼ cup minced shallot

½ cup freshly squeezed orange juice (from 2 oranges)

½ cup water

⅛ teaspoon ground cinnamon

¼ teaspoon kosher salt

1 cup whole-wheat couscous

1. Heat the oil in a saucepan over medium heat. Once the oil is shimmering, add the shallot and cook for 2 minutes, stirring frequently. Add the orange juice, water, cinnamon, and salt, and bring to a boil.

2. Once the liquid is boiling, add the couscous, cover the pan, and turn off the heat. Leave the couscous covered for 5 minutes. When the couscous is done, fluff with a fork.

3. Place ¾ cup of couscous in each of 4 containers.

STORAGE _Store covered containers in the refrigerator for up to 5 days. Freeze for up to 2 months._

TIP _If you have a few extra minutes and want an extra hit of orange flavor, finely zest an orange and add it to the couscous._

Per Serving: Total calories: 215; Total fat: 4g; Saturated fat: <1g; Sodium: 147mg; Carbohydrates: 41g; Fiber: 5g; Protein: 8g

Creamy Polenta *with* Chives *and* Parmesan

MAKES 5 SERVINGS

PREP TIME:
10 minutes

——

COOK TIME:
15 minutes

——

Polenta is an Italian word for a dish that is essentially boiled cornmeal with lots of butter, cream, and cheese. To make this a healthier version, I've substituted white wine, chives, and Parmesan cheese to impart flavor.

1 teaspoon olive oil

¼ cup minced shallot

½ cup white wine

3¼ cups water

¾ cup cornmeal

3 tablespoons grated Parmesan cheese

½ teaspoon kosher salt

¼ cup chopped chives

1. Heat the oil in a saucepan over medium heat. Once the oil is shimmering, add the shallot and sauté for 2 minutes. Add the wine and water and bring to a boil.

2. Pour the cornmeal in a thin, even stream into the liquid, stirring continuously until the mixture starts to thicken.

3. Reduce the heat to low and continue to cook for 10 to 12 minutes, whisking every 1 to 2 minutes.

4. Turn the heat off and stir in the cheese, salt, and chives. Cool.

5. Place about ¾ cup of polenta in each of 5 containers.

STORAGE *Store covered containers in the refrigerator for up to 5 days.*

TIP *When polenta cools, it will take the shape of its container. Once it is reheated, give it a stir, and it will become creamy again.*

Per Serving: Total calories: 110; Total fat: 3g; Saturated fat: 1g; Sodium: 297mg; Carbohydrates: 16g; Fiber: 1g; Protein: 3g

Bulgur Pilaf *with* Almonds

**MAKES
4 SERVINGS**

PREP TIME:
10 minutes

―――

COOK TIME:
20 minutes

―――

Bulgur wheat is one of the easiest whole grains to cook! In fact, you just need to heat the water to boiling, then turn off the stove and allow the bulgur to sit until the water is absorbed. Not only is bulgur a good source of iron, but it's also packed with fiber that may promote good heart and gut health.

⅔ cup uncooked bulgur

1⅓ cups water

¼ cup sliced almonds

1 cup small diced red bell pepper

⅓ cup chopped fresh cilantro

1 tablespoon olive oil

¼ teaspoon salt

1. Place the bulgur and water in a saucepan and bring the water to a boil. Once the water is at a boil, cover the pot with a lid and turn off the heat. Let the covered pot stand for 20 minutes.

2. Transfer the cooked bulgur to a large mixing bowl and add the almonds, peppers, cilantro, oil, and salt. Stir to combine.

3. Place about 1 cup of bulgur in each of 4 containers.

STORAGE *Store covered containers in the refrigerator for up to 5 days. Bulgur can be either reheated or eaten at room temperature.*

TIP *If you don't like cilantro, try another herb. This pilaf is a great way use up herbs you may have in the refrigerator.*

Per Serving: Total calories: 175; Total fat: 7g; Saturated fat: 1g; Sodium: 152mg; Carbohydrates: 25g; Fiber: 6g; Protein: 4g

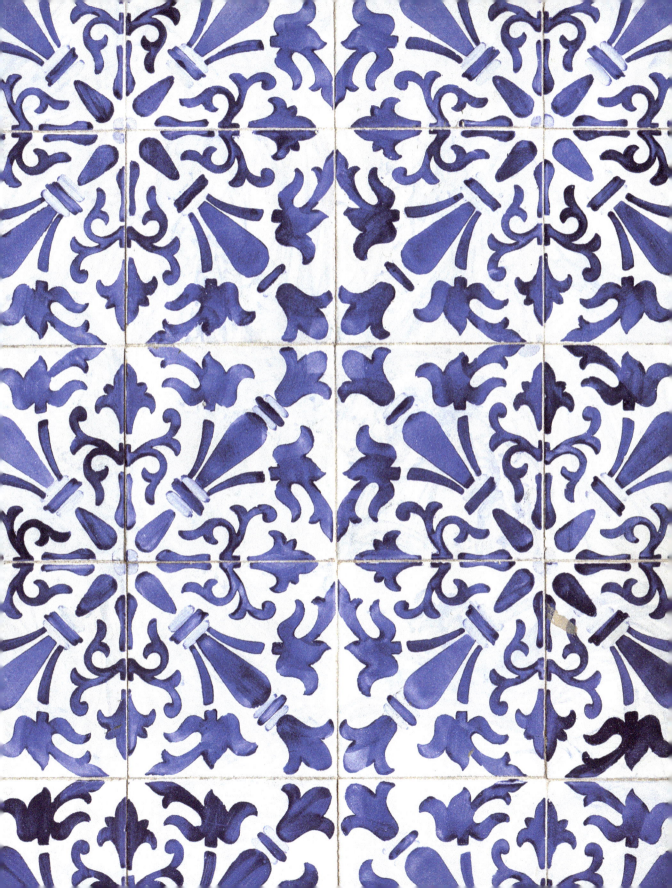

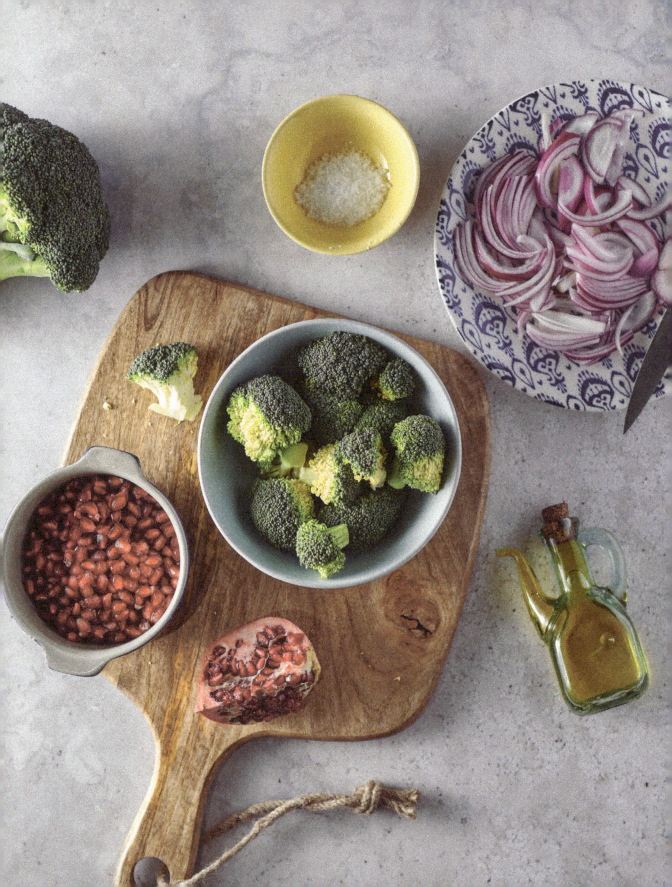

Measurement Conversions

VOLUME EQUIVALENTS (LIQUID)

US Standard	US Standard (ounces)	Metric (approximate)
2 tablespoons	1 fl. oz.	30 mL
¼ cup	2 fl. oz.	60 mL
½ cup	4 fl. oz.	120 mL
1 cup	8 fl. oz.	240 mL
1½ cups	12 fl. oz.	355 mL
2 cups or 1 pint	16 fl. oz.	475 mL
4 cups or 1 quart	32 fl. oz.	1 L
1 gallon	128 fl. oz.	4 L

OVEN TEMPERATURES

Fahrenheit (F)	Celsius (C) (approximate)
250°F	120°C
300°F	150°C
325°F	165°C
350°F	180°C
375°F	190°C
400°F	200°C
425°F	220°C
450°F	230°C

VOLUME EQUIVALENTS (DRY)

US Standard	Metric (approximate)
⅛ teaspoon	0.5 mL
¼ teaspoon	1 mL
½ teaspoon	2 mL
¾ teaspoon	4 mL
1 teaspoon	5 mL
1 tablespoon	15 mL
¼ cup	59 mL
⅓ cup	79 mL
½ cup	118 mL
⅔ cup	156 mL
¾ cup	177 mL
1 cup	235 mL
2 cups or 1 pint	475 mL
3 cups	700 mL
4 cups or 1 quart	1 L

WEIGHT EQUIVALENTS

US Standard	Metric (approximate)
½ ounce	15 g
1 ounce	30 g
2 ounces	60 g
4 ounces	115 g
8 ounces	225 g
12 ounces	340 g
16 ounces or 1 pound	455 g

References

Davis, Courtney, Janet Bryan, Jonathan Hodgson, and Karen Murphy. "Definition of the Mediterranean Diet: A Literature Review." *Nutrients* 7, no. 11 (November 2015): 9139–53.

Martinez-Gonzalez, Miguel A., Jordi Salas-Salvado, Ramón Estruch, Dolores Corella, Montse Fitó, and Emilio Ros. "Benefits of the Mediterranean Diet: Insights from the PREDIMED Study." *Progress in Cardiovascular Diseases* 58, no. 1 (July–August 2015): 50–60.

Tosti, Valeria, Beatrice Bertozzi, and Luigi Fontana. "Health Benefits of the Mediterranean Diet: Metabolic and Molecular Mechanisms." *Journals of Gerontology: Series A* 73, no. 3 (March 2018): 318–26.

Index

Acknowledgments

My husband, Ramin Oskoui, deserves a giant thank-you for putting up with my crazy schedule during the preparation of this book and for supporting me through his words of encouragement, positivity, and of course being my main taste tester. I couldn't have done this without him.

I wouldn't have arrived at this point in my career without the support of parents who probably thought I would be a professional student for a good portion of my life! I think most parents would probably have gotten upset when their 19-year-old child spent the summer working at Disneyland and then decided to drop out of college and move to Seattle for culinary school. Thanks, Mom, for putting up with my mess in the kitchen from elementary school through high school! Thank you to the Oskoui side of my family for always showing their support and encouragement to help me reach great heights.

Thanks to my USC Hospitality family for always supporting my extracurricular activities. I told a few of you in 2018 that I wanted to write a cookbook, and who knew that intention would be fulfilled one year later?

A big shout-out to my editor Gurvinder Gandu for walking me through this intense book process for my first time, and to Sal Taymuree for giving me this opportunity.

About the Author

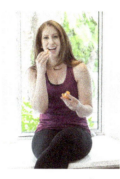

LINDSEY PINE, MS, RDN, CLT, is the owner of Tasty Balance Nutrition, specializing in recipe development and nutrition communications supporting a heart-healthy lifestyle. In addition to writing for her own blog, she has contributed to numerous publications, including *Reader's Digest, Self, Today's Dietitian,* and *Campus Dining Today.*

Lindsey is also the Dining Dietitian for USC Hospitality on the campus of the University of Southern California. Her education includes a culinary degree from Seattle Central Community College, a bachelor's degree in hospitality and tourism management from San Diego State University, and a master's degree in nutritional science from Cal State Los Angeles.

She and her husband currently reside in her hometown of Los Angeles.

CPSIA information can be obtained
at www.ICGtesting.com
Printed in the USA
JSHW011342210420
5206JS00002B/2

9 781646 115020